Maladies and Medicine

Maladies and Medicine

Exploring Health and Healing
1540–1740

Jennifer Evans and Sara Read

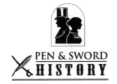

PEN & SWORD
HISTORY

First published in Great Britain in 2017 by
Pen & Sword History
an imprint of
Pen & Sword Books Ltd
47 Church Street
Barnsley
South Yorkshire
S70 2AS

ISBN 978 1 47387 571 5

Printed and bound in Malta by Gutenberg Press Ltd.

Pen & Sword Books Ltd incorporates the Imprints of Pen & Sword Books
Archaeology, Atlas, Aviation, Battleground, Discovery, Family History, History,
Maritime, Military, Naval, Politics, Railways, Select, Transport, True Crime,
Fiction, Frontline Books, Leo Cooper, Praetorian Press, Seaforth Publishing,
Wharncliffe and White Owl.

For a complete list of Pen & Sword titles please contact
PEN & SWORD BOOKS LIMITED
47 Church Street, Barnsley, South Yorkshire, S70 2AS, England
E-mail: enquiries@pen-and-sword.co.uk
Website: www.pen-and-sword.co.uk

Contents

Acknowledgements   vii
Introduction   viii

PART ONE   HEAD COMPLAINTS   1

Chapter 1   Migraine and Headache: A Laborious and Dull Sense   2
Chapter 2   Epilepsy: The Sacred Disease   10
Chapter 3   Palsy: Paralysis or Shaking   17
Chapter 4   Eye Complaints: Light without Heat   23
Chapter 5   Toothache: Rotten Worms   30

PART TWO   ABDOMINAL MALADIES   37

Chapter 6   Disorderly Bowels: Griping Guts   38
Chapter 7   Jaundice: Shedding Choler   43
Chapter 8   Kidney and Bladder Stones: Easing the Passage   50

PART THREE WHOLE BODY AILMENTS   59

Chapter 9   Agues: Frequent Fits of Fever   60
Chapter 10 Cancer: In the Crab's Claws   67
Chapter 11 Diabetes: The Pissing Evil   73
Chapter 12 Dropsy: Drowning in Water   79
Chapter 13 Gout: A Painful Guest   84
Chapter 14 Irritating Infestations: Rubbing and Scratching   91
Chapter 15 Pestilential Plague: A Divine Affliction   98
Chapter 16 Scrofula: The King's Evil   107
Chapter 17 Scurvy: Scabs, Spots, and Stinking Breath   113
Chapter 18 Smallpox: Red Pustules and Scarlet Cloth   119

PART FOUR   REPRODUCTIVE MALADIES   127

Chapter 19 Greensickness: The Virgin's Disease   128
Chapter 20 The Whites: A Most Troublesome Disease   133

Chapter 21   Infertility: A Defect in the Seed   138
Chapter 22   False Conceptions and Miscarriages: Breeding Moles   143
Chapter 23   Venereal Disease: The French Pox, a New Disease   152

Afterword   161
List of Illustrations   162
Bibliography   166
Index   179

Acknowledgements

This book is a product of the shared passion we have for all things to do with medicine and the body in the early modern era. It has been a joy to research and write and has taught us one or two new things along the way.

We met when we were both awarded postdoctoral fellowships by the Society for Renaissance Studies, and so will always be grateful to the Society for the awards and for facilitating a fruitful partnership. We would like to thank our colleagues at Loughborough University and the University of Hertfordshire.

The illustrations that bring this medical story to life are reproduced courtesy of the generosity of the Wellcome Images collection and the Rijksmuseum, who offer many of their digital images under creative commons licences or in the public domain. Their generosity is greatly appreciated.

Finally we would like to thank our friends and family for their constant support of our endeavours and their enthusiasm for our work. Particular thanks go to Maximillian Dupenois, Pete Read, and George Wiltshire.

This book is dedicated to the memory of William Johnston (1930-2016).

A Note on the Original Texts

Some quotations from early modern texts have been modernised to make the sense accessible while retaining the original meaning. Certain titles of these texts have also been regularised in the book on the same basis, but all appear in their original form in the bibliography.

Introduction

'Live Well, die never; Die well, live ever'

– Sarah Wigges

As the inscription on the commonplace book belonging to Sarah Wigges, compiled in 1616, suggests, healthcare in early modern times was a holistic business. All sorts of factors worked together to produce optimum health, including diet, exercise, and faith. Underpinning all these factors were the medical theories of ancient writers such as the Greek medic Hippocrates, often called the father of modern medicine, Roman physician Claudius Galen, and Aristotle. The Hippocratic writings are now known to have been written by a group of people rather than by one man, and this collection of medical writing influenced medical practice for 2,000 years. Hippocratic medicine imagined the human body worked by way of a fluid exchange. These bodily fluids, known as humours, needed to be kept in balance to maintain health. All fluid elements in the body were known as humours, so that for example, the fluids in the eye are still named the aqueous and vitreous humour.

There were thought to be four main liquids or humours in the body, and it was believed these were connected to the four elements of the earth. Blood was related to air and spring; yellow bile (choler) was related to fire and summer; black bile (melancholy) was related to the earth and autumn; and phlegm was related to water and winter. Under this system someone's personality was linked to their humoral makeup, so it would be assumed that someone quick to anger would naturally have too much yellow bile in their body. Similarly, the symptoms of what we would think of today as depression were linked to having too much melancholy in the system and steps would be taken to rebalance the humours of people diagnosed as melancholic. The connection of these bodily and personality features to the humours was all encompassing. John Fage's book *Speculum Ægrotorum*, published in 1606, demonstrates this by providing detailed descriptions of the different humoral constitutions. For instance, Fage explained that choleric men were 'for the most part' short because their natural heat destroyed and consumed the 'natural moisture' necessary for growth, they sooner had beards, were naturally quick-witted, courageous and had strong appetites.

However, they were also liable to be arrogant, graceless, quarrelsome, fraudulent, inconstant and crafty. By contrast, melancholic men lacked natural heat and so were tall of stature and slender of body. They had little hair, were pale and were often without beards. Their personality tended to be studious, timorous, stubborn and fretful. Phlegmatic men, hindered by their body's overabundance of cold wet humours, were likely to be shorter, 'gross & fat', without hair or beards. They were slothful, forgetful, cowardly, covetous, and vain. Finally, sanguine men, whose bodies abounded with blood, were, in Fage's opinion, 'men of middle form, their bodies are well composed, with large limbs, fleshy, but not fat, with great veins & arteries, with smooth skins, and hot and moist in feeling, the body hairy and soon bearded.' These men were merciful, courteous, bold, lecherous, trusty and faithful.

Balancing humours, within the natural innate characteristics of an individual's constitution, was considered fundamental to health. Physicians and others sought to rebalance the humours of unwell people by many means, such as controlling their diets, so phlegmatic patients might be prescribed a 'drying' diet, for example. More drastic but routine interventions included administering emetics to induce vomiting, cupping or scarification to draw malign humours out through the skin, or even drawing blood by means of a small incision, or the use of leeches. Blood was universally understood to have two origins: the heart and the liver. The heart, brain, and liver together were what Galen called the 'noble organs'. This changed in the 1620s when William Harvey, physician at the Stuart court, conducted a series of experiments on live animals to prove that in fact the body had one circulation system. Blood was produced in the liver and pumped around the body. However, although his findings were published as *Exercitatio Anatomica de Motu Cordis et Sanguinis in Animalibus* (1628), the new theory took a while to be integrated into medical practices and the true implications of Harvey's work only became known years later. As late as 1682, physician Thomas Gibson mentioned in his book, *The Anatomy of Human Bodies Epitomized*, that he supposed doctors must accept the theory of circulation as true. Part of the reason for the slow integration of this radical new knowledge was the influence the ancient medics held. Empirical (evidence-based) knowledge had to find a place within the existing truisms before being accepted.

Gendered Bodies: Women

In the humoral system, women's bodies were thought to be colder and wetter than the male hot and dry body. To understand the situation of the female sexual organs, Galen asked readers to visualise 'Turn[ing] outwardly the woman's, turn inward so to speak, and fold double the man's, and you will find them the same in both every respect.' This worked in a culture that relied on visual metaphors to aid understanding, but didn't mean that people thought that male and female bodies worked in identical ways.

One key to understanding women's bodies was through the effects of her womb. In a famous letter reputedly sent to Hippocrates in ancient Greece, and often quoted in early modern medical texts, the womb was described as being the 'cause of six hundred miseries, and innumerable Calamities.' Also in accordance with Hippocratic writings, and at least until the seventeenth century, some people claimed that the womb could actually move around the body, causing feelings of suffocation as it pressed against the diaphragm. Galen did not subscribe to this belief, but it still held sway. Some ancient writers even described the womb as being like a wild animal inside the female body.

Another facet of the coolness of women's bodies was that it was assumed that they were looser and more prone to leaking than the firmer, drier male body. Medical norms also presumed that women led more sedate lives than men, and so they didn't use up all their blood in the way that men did, necessitating menstruation. Likewise, their sedate lives and inefficient use of the food they consumed meant that women put down more fat than men. That women didn't normally menstruate when pregnant was because the body used the usually surplus blood nourishing the infant. After birth, this blood was redirected to breasts where an innate facility there concocted it into milk.

Gendered Bodies: Men

Women's bodies in this era were clearly distinguished by unique physiological processes and by the central role the womb played in their experience of health and illness. In contrast to this it has been said that men's bodies were the 'perfect' or 'normal' constant against which women's bodies were compared. Yet to think in such ways obscures the full picture. Men obviously suffered from sickness and disease and their bodies were not inevitably, or always, perfect and normal. Indeed, Stephen Hobbs asked in 1610: 'For what is Man, if he have not his health?' He noted that men suffered from gout, bladder and kidney stones, ulcers in the bladder, tumours and swellings, hernias, and fistulas as well as fractures and dislocations. The diseases Hobbs listed were experienced by both sexes, but some had developed a common association with the male body. Gout, as we will see, was considered a masculine disease, as were bladder stones (as one advantage of women's softer, more 'leaky', bodies was that they were thought to pass stones more easily, rendering them relatively free from the condition). The early modern male body was considered to be hot and dry which, while admirable, did make it prone to certain disorders. Moreover, several medical writers of the early modern period acknowledged and investigated conditions that afflicted the male reproductive and sexual organs including phimosis, a narrowing of the foreskin, and impotence. While conditions like infertility were not restricted to one sex, medical writers were clear that even when the same causes might be to blame, such conditions could manifest in clearly gendered ways.

Men's bodily complexion was thought to be manifest in their distinct physiology. Their complexions gave a physical basis for their superior rationality and the presence of their muscular tissue, a more vehement pulse and a strong, deep voice. Scholars have viewed men's bodies as an important foundation for seventeenth-century notions of manhood and household patriarchy. While the ownership of a male body did not necessarily confer these qualities, the attainment of such power did, in part, rest on the display of a well-formed, moderately-strong, virile body. Importantly men's ability to control and discipline their bodies demonstrated their superiority in the social hierarchy. Men's bodies were therefore not supposed to leak or be disrupted by excessive eating, drinking, or sexual activity. Nonetheless, men did suffer from incontinence, gleet (a shedding of seminal matter), and haemorrhoids, all of which undermined this ideal of bodily control.

Culpeper's Neutral Health

Nowadays we tend to think of ourselves as either well or ill, although many of us would acknowledge that we live with little niggles of pain or sensations of bodily discomfort. In the seventeenth century things were no different. The Galenic text the *Ars Medica* had been an important part of university curricula for physicians since the thirteenth century, and it spoke of three bodily conditions – the healthy, the ill, and the neutral. Neutral bodies were those such as the infirm, the elderly, and those recovering from ill health. In its origins, neutrality was a philosophical concept, however into the sixteenth century it was linked to ideas of complexion and became much more important for diagnosis. In this new form it also came to mean a body with a balanced temperament.

It is unclear how far physicians actually employed the idea of neutral bodies in their medical practice, but it has been suggested that the idea of a neutral body was more often deployed in discussions about ageing. In this case the body was not always in a state of health, as it had been in youth, but was also not always diseased. Therefore neutral was a useful category for discussing bodily conditions that fell outside of the remit of therapeutic medicine. By the seventeenth century neutral was no longer being used as a diagnostic tool, and the neutral body became less relevant to practitioners who were much more focused on therapeutics, and indeed on understanding the ageing process.

Instead, neutrality became a term used to describe illness and bodily states that medical practitioners couldn't deal with, particularly with the introduction of new medical ideas based on mechanics and hydraulics, which were promoted in the later seventeenth century. Nevertheless, Nicholas Culpeper still related the concept to his readership. In his translation of *Galen's Art of Physick*, he claimed that a healthy body was simply 'when it is in good natural temper'. An unhealthy body was one that suffered from what we would consider a congenital birth defect, or one that was 'at present sick [...] or distemper'd in mind, [...] broken or bruised'. Finally, the neutral body was 'an exquisite medium between healthful and unhealthful'. Culpeper claimed that people in this condition were '*neither sick enough to lie in Bed, nor well enough to follow his Employment*'. A modern comparison might be the experience of a mild cold, which is often considered very annoying, but not enough to disrupt daily life.

Natural Requirements for Health

As has been outlined, the healthy body was thought to depend on a balance of its humours. The humours were one of the seven 'naturals', as Culpeper in his translation of Galen said, required for health. The others were spirits, elements, complexions, members, virtues and operations; along with humours, these were things that made up the natural body.

Non-natural Factors

Throughout the era covered by this book men and women not only responded to bouts of ill-health, but also attempted to preserve their health. They focused as much on preventative medicine as they did therapeutics. A key part of both preventative medicine and therapeutics was maintaining a healthy 'regimen' by regulating the six non-naturals. These were not 'unnatural' elements, but were things that affected the body – air, food and drink, motion and rest, sleep and waking, repletion and evacuation (including sexual emissions), and emotions or passions. Health was, therefore, much like the modern day, connected to a close monitoring and regulation of daily life. Understanding these elements created an easily accessible and flexible means to take active steps in the prevention of disease. The flexibility of the framework was useful because these factors would affect different bodily constitutions in different ways, therefore people had to focus their efforts in different ways.

According to the Stars: Therapeutic Astrology

'I always found the Disease vary according to the various motion of the Stars, and this is enough one would think to teach a man by the Effect where the Cause lay', wrote Nicholas Culpeper. And as this statement implies, he believed that the heavens exerted a definable influence over the body and health in this era. In his *pharmacopoeias* or lists of remedies, he outlined the virtues of herbs and how these related to the planets that had dominion over them. So, for example, in a posthumous edition of *The English Physician Enlarged* from 1669, readers were informed that '*Mars* owns' barberries and 'presents it to the use of my Country-men to purge their bodies of Choler'. The mulberry tree, meanwhile, was ruled by Mercury and so its 'effects [were] variable as his are'.

Astrology was not looked upon in the early part of this period as a superstitious practice but as an acceptable art form practiced by many famous men, including John Dee, astrologer to Elizabeth I. Astrologers were called upon to cast horoscopes to answer a range of questions about family relationships, potential marriages, journeys, and investments. Ben Jonson's play *The Alchemist* (1610) has one tobacco retailer, Abel Drugger, consult the eponymous chemical physician for astrological advice on matters ranging from the best days to close deals, to the arrangement of shelves in his new premises.

Astrological medicine, as Culpeper's comments suggest, was based upon the premise that parts of the body were governed by different star signs. Scorpio governed the genitalia and reproductive organs, while Aries dictated illnesses of the head. The association of particular star signs with particular bodily functions and parts appears to have been arbitrary. This rather haphazard attribution was noted by some at the time. William Rowland wrote in his book *Judicall Astrologie, Judicially Condemned* (1652), that 'the government of the Signs of the body is not taken from experience in nature, but feigned long ago by some drowsy pate, and now because it hath a cloak of antiquity, it is allowed.' As just one rational argument in his favour, he said it was contradictory to associate Aries, which was a hot sign, with the brain, which in the humoral model was characterised as cold. Different types of illness were also explained in relation to the qualities of heavenly bodies. Acute diseases were linked with the moon, which was changeable and unstable. Melancholy was associated with Saturn because it was dim and slow moving.

Astrological medical practitioners would cast horoscopes based on the moment a disease had struck a patient (or if this was unknown, the time from which they were confined to bed). The horoscope would reveal the type, severity and prognosis of the disease and would allow the practitioner to offer a prescription for medication. While this practice was criticised by some for being inaccurate, both Simon Forman and Richard Napier ran successful medical practices based on these methods. Napier, a dour clergyman, spent forty years tending to the bodies and souls of his Buckinghamshire flock. He treated a range of ailments and conditions including madness. Overall though, the popularity of astrological medicine waned throughout this era.

God, Christianity and Cures

The humoral model, problematically, was fundamentally pagan, created by men who did not follow the Christian faith. This caused some consternation for early modern men and women, but did not form a fundamental barrier to adopting the framework. Rather, throughout the period, humoral theory was integrated with Christian beliefs. Moreover, Christianity was seen as a healing religion: Christ, after all, healed those who were sick in body and in mind.

Healing the body and maintaining its health was also a religious imperative because the body was the house of the immortal soul, but by contrast, enduring ill-health bravely was thought to be a way of becoming more spiritual. It provided a trial of faith, or an experience that facilitated reflection on one's own life and actions. It was also universally believed that God was the primary source of all illness and disease. Adam and Eve had brought disease into the world at the moment of the Fall and each person's individual illnesses were dictated by God's will. Particularly in the post-Reformation Protestant fervour, illness was read as a sign of God's providence and men and women scrutinised their bodily condition for signs of salvation. As well as afflicting mankind with disease, God had provided healing substances, particularly in the form of plants, which were to be used to heal the body. However, these were unlikely to work if a patient had not sufficiently repented of the behaviour that had caused them to be struck down in the first place. Medicines were believed to work only once God had allowed them to, thus prayer was an important part of most healing regimes; medicine and prayer went hand in glove and people were expected to seek medical help for their illnesses. Physicians and healers did not always emphasise the importance of prayer in their writings as it had the potential to undermine their own usefulness, but many of them did acknowledge God in their case notes. For example, Stratford-upon-Avon based physician John Hall, son-in-law of the playwright William Shakespeare, routinely noted how he cured a patient with conventional medicines, but gave the ultimate credit to God for the return to health of his patient.

For some medical practitioners the irreligious nature of the humoral model was much more problematic. The German-Swiss Renaissance physician Theophrastus Aurelius von Hohenheim, self-styled Paracelsus (because his skills surpassed those of first century BCE Roman medical writer Aulus Cornelius Celsus), set out to create a truly Christian medical framework. Paracelsus was a rather controversial figure even in his own lifetime. Yet after his death in 1541, and particularly in the 1550s, his medical ideas became much more influential. In 1575, a two-volume collection of twenty-six of his treatises was published and by the end of the century, editor Johannes Huser could boast of printing a ten-volume definitive collection of Paracelsian works.

Alongside this mass of publication, more and more medical practitioners were claiming to follow his new 'chemical ideas'. In 1585, R. Bostocke claimed that the 'great number of learned Philosophers and Physicians, as well as were Galenists, as others, which at this day do embrace, follow and practise, the doctrine, methods and ways of curing of this Chemical Physick.' This new Christian medicine proposed that the cosmos was composed of three active substances: mercury, which was transformative; sulphur, which was binding; and salt, which was stabilising. Ill health in this new model was the result of dysfunctional chemical processes in the body. A rather more radical idea, when compared to the humoral model, was the idea that diseases were specific entities that would afflict different people in the same way.

As suggested here, many people adopted Paracelsus's ideas, but one particularly influential man was the Flemish physician Jean Baptist van Helmont who was born in 1579. He read and admired Paracelsus's new ideas, but felt that he had made some errors. Like other chemical physicians he argued that chemical reactions were central to understanding the body, particularly fermentation, effervescence, and putrefaction. Digestion, for example, was explained as a process of fermentation that occurred in the stomach.

The centrality of Christian doctrine to this new body of medical thought meant that some people saw chemical practitioners as more accessible and more charitable than their Galenic counterparts. Chemical physicians were also some of the first to criticise the practice of bloodletting. Helmontians, followers of van Helmont, not only argued that phlebotomy weakened the body, but that it embodied the cruelty and dispassion of Galenic healers. Bloodletting cut into the body and drained its life force. The Bible clearly stated that life was connected to the blood, it was not something to be coldly counted and calculated by uncaring physicians as it was drained from the body of the sick and vulnerable. Several writers launched vituperative attacks on this practice, one argued that it was 'an inhumane barbarous butchery, because so much blood as is taken away, so much is cut off from the thread of life [...] cutting short the life of many by the rules of his Art, or at least impairing their strength.'

In the 1660s clashes between chemical physicians who tended to be self-taught healers interested in chemical experimentation – although they did have several well-respected physicians amongst their ranks – and university-educated traditional physicians came to a head. Led by practitioners such as Thomas O'Dowde, a courtier of Charles II, iatrochemists (as they were sometimes known) pressed for a royal charter to legitimise their work and bring it to parity with the doctors admitted to the Royal College of Physicians. The College vehemently opposed this, claiming that the apothecaries (the pharmacists of their day) had a guild with which the chemical physicians should seek to merge. As late as 1674 Mary Trye, O'Dowde's daughter, issued a direct challenge to Henry Stubbe, author of *An Epistolary Discourse Concerning Phlebotomy* (1671), that she could cure people of prevalent diseases like smallpox much more proficiently with her chemical 'methods and medicines' than he ever could through bloodletting. Chemical medicine never got its royal charter, despite its long history of royal patronage, and waned as a discrete discipline largely because its effective cures were incorporated into traditional medicine and the source of the ferments in the body were never located.

Mechanical medical theories, mentioned above, also grew up at this time. These were based on physics and supported by eminent physicians.

They sought to understand the muscular system in mechanical ways, but also incorporated new ways of thinking about the hydraulic exchange of humoralism. They suggested mechanical models for some chemical processes. Instead of digestion being due to chemical ferment it was caused by pulverizing and churning. A key figure in this field was Santorio Sanctorius; born of noble parents, he received his medical degree from Padua in 1582 aged just 21. Italian physician Lorenzo Bellini also created a theory about hydraulic iatromechanism, adopted in Scotland by James Keill and in England by Stephen Hales. Archibald Pitcairne, a physician in Edinburgh, refined this model and argued that the body was a series of canals in which fluids circulated. He linked Newton's ideas about gravity and its effects on the tides, to ideas about pressures of fluids in vessels within the body. Despite holding a chair in chemistry at Oxford University, Dr John Freind, author of the first monograph on menstruation, *Emmenologia* published in 1703, used Pitcairne's Newtonian ideas to explain this function. In the eighteenth century, after the span of this book, both of these ideas would be overtaken by ideas about nerves and sensibilities, building on work begun in the late seventeenth century by Oxford based physician Thomas Willis.

Empiricism and Experimentation

As well as the rise of chemical medicine and mechanical theories, another change was occurring in this era. Initially physicians and medical practitioners revered Galenic medicine and ancient theory. University medical training was largely a matter of learning these ancient scripts, and so attempts to bolster a reputation would focus on the healer's familiarity with the works of Galen, Hippocrates, and Aristotle. Increasingly throughout the era this gave way to the rise of empiricism. The notion that experimentation and, more importantly, experience, underpinned a practitioner's therapeutic practices. Thus, for example, Simon Mason could argue in the preface of his 1745 book on intermitting fevers that his considerable practice at St Andrews' hospital for the poor in Holborn made him the most suitable healer to advise people on the nature and treatment of the disease. He claimed:

> *While some have been at their Books, in Search after the Nature of Distempers, and their Cures, I have been attending the Sick; observing strictly the Nature of the Disease, and the Indications of the various Symptoms and their Tendencies, waiting the Effects of Medicines, and from long Practice, Observations, and Reflections [...] to confirm the*

Notions I had long indulged, in Relation to the Nature of Intermitting Fevers and Agues.

To drive home his point he argued:

SUPPOSE *two Persons of the same Capacity, the one read all the Accounts, he could meet with, of the* East Indies, *the other should go over, and take all the Notice he could, and by seeing and conversing with the Natives, observing their Customs, Habits, Manners, Religions, &c. every one will agree, the last is the Person to be relied on, for the Exactness of his Account.*

Mason was not the first, and certainly was not the last, to make such arguments. Handbills printed throughout the seventeenth century, designed to advertise the services of unlicensed practitioners also emphasised their experience and empiricism. Both men and women used this trope. One advertisement for a 'Gentlewoman' operating in Exeter Street in the Strand claimed that her remedies worked because of God's blessing and her 'diligent experience in Physick and Chirurgery for more than 20 years past'. The midwife Jane Sharp conceded that some theoretical learning was necessary, but wrote in her 1671 midwifery manual that it was not 'hard words' that did the work but years of hands–on practice.

In a small part, the work of Francis Bacon, writing in the early seventeenth century on natural philosophy, influenced this change. He proposed a new method for studying the natural world, one that would require men to radically change the way in which they perceived knowledge and learning. Rather than seeing science as a contemplation and organisation of pre-existing truths, he wanted it to be an endeavour to create knowledge, the discovery of the unknown. He proposed these ideas in his tome on natural philosophy, *Novum Organum* (1620). Observation and experiment were key to this, as was the ability to measure accurately, something that was becoming ever more possible with the invention and development of a range of new scientific instruments. Bacon's belief that scientific enquiry would help to improve mankind's experiences and ease suffering, was particularly influential in the mid-seventeenth century during the turbulence of the republican experiment. The foundation of the Royal Society after the Restoration helped cement these principles and fostered the collaboration he had also called for. Later again, in the eighteenth century, French philosophers emphasised his works and ideas as a means of promoting scientific endeavour.

Hierarchy of Health Professionals

The sick of early modern England did not have the luxury of national healthcare provided free at point of contact. Instead they turned to a range of practitioners who operated in what has come to be called the medical marketplace. This term is rather problematic for some historians because it foregrounds economics in the practice of healthcare. Despite this concern though, it neatly encapsulates the complex and mixed medical landscape that patients navigated. The marketplace was composed of what we might call 'professionals', as well as a plethora of 'irregular' (unlicensed), itinerant, magical, and charitable healers, both men and women.

This notion of a medical marketplace replaced the traditional view, somewhat perpetuated by physicians of the time, that medical practice in this era was based on a tripartite model. In this framework three 'professional' groups operated within strict limitations. Physicians who trained at university and acquired a classical education based on Galenic medical theory and attending some anatomical dissections, surgeons who completed an apprenticeship and applied their hands to the body to cure external complaints, and apothecaries, the lowliest in the triangle, whose apprenticeships readied them for making up the prescriptions given to patients by physicians. Yet historians have been unable to identity this system operating clearly in England, and of course it overlooks another important source of healthcare –home remedies or 'kitchen-physic' known to every housewife, which was in reality the first port of call for most people.

Bishops around the country provided licenses to surgeons, physicians and midwives. The Royal College of Physicians (established in 1518 and granted a royal charter in 1523) attempted to maintain a monopoly over medical practice in London by regulating physicians and practitioners within a seven-mile radius of the city. Historians, particularly Margaret Pelling, have shown that the college pursued a range of practitioners who operated without licences. They were not able to successfully maintain a monopoly however, thus allowing for the thriving medical marketplace to develop in London, and across the country. One reason why non-licentiate practitioners flourished was that many people simply could not afford the services of a physician, who tended to be rather costly. Another reason was that people would seek the advice of multiple healers; this might include a physician, but also included other practitioners as well.

Throughout the early modern era, surgeons pushed against the notion that they were less prestigious than physicians because of the difference in their education and the fact that they worked with their hands. They were sometimes denigrated for the fact that they did 'manual' labour on the body and that they handled diseased and dirty bodies on a regular basis. This was perhaps reinforced by the fact that their guild was the barber-surgeons guild, formed since barbers performed minor surgery like tooth-drawing, skills that were initially seen as allied. The Barbers' Company was formed in the fifteenth century and the Fellowship of Surgeons joined it in 1540, in an Act of Union passed by King Henry VIII. Because their work required manual labour and theoretical knowledge, surgeons were able to shape their identity as both learned and as artisanal. Some could therefore claim that they were the preeminent healers of the day because they could do everything a physician could do, and in addition could practice surgery – a physician, they argued, was a lesser practitioner because they could not carry out surgical cures.

Another shift that occurred during the era was that apothecaries became much more than just drug dispensers. In the theory of the tripartite system they were only supposed to produce the prescriptions given by physicians, and were often disparaged as poor, low-grade dispensers of risky remedies. The term 'apothecary' came from the word 'apotheca', the name for a place where wine, herbs and spices were stored. It was originally used to describe people who kept and sold these commodities. It is therefore unsurprising that apothecaries were originally part of the company of Grocers (est. 1428). It wasn't until 1617 that James I created the Worshipful Society of Apothecaries by royal charter. He explained that he had split the trades because grocers were 'but merchants', while the trade of the apothecary required much more skill and knowledge. In many cases, apothecaries diagnosed patients and offered their own prescriptions and treatment ideas. Richard Wiseman, surgeon in ordinary to Charles II, recorded in his book *Several Chirurgical Treatises* (1686) the case of one patient treated by a group including himself, a physician, and an apothecary. The patient lodged in the apothecary's house for the duration of his treatment. When his recovery progressed slower than anticipated, Wiseman questioned the patient and discovered that the apothecary had altered the dosage of the prescribed medication. When confronted on this issue, Wiseman claimed that the apothecary was unrepentant and continued to defy the supposedly more prestigious surgeon and physician. By the eighteenth century apothecaries were actively redefining their role and were becoming more explicitly 'doctors', or what we might think of as a general practitioner.

There was much variation in attitude and practice amongst these 'professional' groups, and patients sought out different practitioners and healers in different circumstances. In the past it has been assumed that, outside of urban areas, access to physicians was limited. However, Ian Mortimer has re-evaluated this picture and revealed that in the south of England people did have access to physicians if they wanted to consult them. In reality however, many people would seek assistance from the women they knew before calling upon the services of these professional healers. According to the famous guide for housewives, Gervase Markham's *The English Housewife* (1625), one of a woman's primary roles as a wife and mistress of the house was to provide medical care for those in her charge. Thus it was the lady of the manor who tended to her family, household, and tenants on her estates. These women often had access to large kitchen gardens and the distilleries needed to make treatments such as decoctions from distilled herbs. Elizabethan noblewoman Lady Margaret Hoby, who was often in poor health herself, noted several occasions when she provided medical care, such as in August 1599 when she was called at six in the morning to help 'a wife in travail [labour]', with whom she stayed until she was safely delivered that afternoon. More remarkably, in July 1601 Lady Margaret operated on an infant. The child was born with no 'fundament' or anal opening, so had 'no passage for excrements but at the mouth'. Despite her best attempts, cutting deeply and searching the child internally she couldn't locate the child's rectal passage. These women could develop reputations for their abilities and people might seek them out for particular treatments, so in June 1631 Sir Gilbert Gerard wrote to Lady Joan Barrington on behalf of a 'poor man' whose son had developed a swelling on his 'cods' (testicles). He wrote to her because his wife remembered that she had 'cured a child at Kingston of such a disease.'

Common Diseases

In 1649 Nicholas Culpeper translated the Royal College of Physicians' medicine guide, the *Pharmacopoeia Londinesis* and published it as *A Physical Directory; or a Translation of the London Dispensatory*. Culpeper's motives were to take control away from the medical elite and into the hands of ordinary people. Until his death, he translated and published many English medical texts, and his reputation was such that in the years following his death works came out ascribed to him, or with him at least as co-translator, along with people such as Abdiah Cole. In 1652 he produced a version of this book called *The English Physician* in which he listed herbs and plants that were available widely and cheaply in England, rather than some of the exotic treatments physicians recommended. Culpeper was sceptical about how much university-educated, elite doctors cared about healing their patients, and how much they practised for the wealth they could accrue. In a barbed comment on such people, Culpeper wrote:

> *Although all men, in Knowledge take delight,*
> *Yet they love money better, that's the spite.*

Reading this book gives an insight into many of the illnesses that Culpeper treated as an apothecary. Many of these diseases or complaints are familiar to us today, but some have long since ceased to be recognised. Culpeper lists cures for asthma, loss of appetite, cancers, coughs and colds, diabetes, headaches, haemorrhoids, jaundice, joint pain, leprosy, lethargy, measles, memory loss, miscarriage, pain, sciatica, shingles, toothache, warts, weight-loss, and wind. Diseases that might be less familiar to a modern reader, but were evidently common enough to warrant a prescription include the falling sickness, King's Evil, morphew, purples, quartan and quotidian agues, pissing blood, quinsy, reds, rheum, running of the reins, spleen, strangury, swooning, watching, and whites. Some of these are, in fact, familiar conditions known by another name, such as 'watching' known today as insomnia, for example. Culpeper listed these conditions alongside entries for what to do if you suspected yourself to be a victim of witchcraft, were suffering from longings, or lechery, or even just wanted to get rid of your freckles.

Causes of Death: Bills of Mortality

One way of getting a picture of what early modern people commonly died from, or thought they were dying from, is through the published Bills of Mortality. These leaflets were produced mainly in London and until the Victorian era. They were published lists of how many people had died in a given week, categorised by what they died from. Although most people bought these leaflets from booksellers at the time as a single sheet, some were collated and then published as a large volume. One such volume published in 1759 brought together the bills covering the period from 1657 to 1758. This 1759 edition offers a history of these documents and suggests that the earliest known bill dates from 1538 but that they appeared intermittently unless they were needed in certain circumstances; the plague outbreaks of the 1590s, for example, necessitated regular bills to keep citizens abreast of the situation. Plague was a very common cause of death at regular points throughout the era, but this particular decade was also a time of shortage and famine. It was the duty of the parish clerk to collate the information, and then the total figure was given for each parish before the breakdown. In the plague year 1593, the parish of St Katherine Coleman recorded 444 deaths, exactly half of which were attributed to the plague. In St Mary Aldermanbury, the proportion of plague victims was higher with fifty-four out of seventy-nine deaths being put down to the disease. To put this into proportion, 17,844 people were buried in London and its Liberties – the area around London under the administrative control of statesmen from within the City walls – of whom 10,662 died of plague; not a single parish declared itself free from the pestilence. Tellingly, only 4,021 infants were christened that year, so the population would have fallen. During the 1590s, the population of London is thought to have risen to around 150,000 people, although exact figures aren't known.

In non-plague years, some of the most common causes of death were fevers and consumptions. In 1680 for example, no one was thought to have died of plague – the last great plague was in 1665 and so this is to be expected, although the threat of the disease meant that it was still listed in the totals. In 1680, 21,053 Londoners died, 11,039 men and 10,014 women. Of these, fevers accounted for over 3,000 souls, with consumption and convulsions being the next most common causes of death. These three conditions accounted for almost half of the deaths. In the same year, 315 women died in childbirth, and 615 stillborn infants were included in the overall figure. The least common causes of death were starvation, from which just one person died, another person died of a headache (which was differentiated from the five who died of megrim (migraine)), and one other died of leprosy; three people were found dead in the street from unknown causes. A shocking eighty-nine infants were reported to have been 'overlain' (accidentally smothered) in bed; sixty-five accidental deaths were noted, along with twenty-three suicides, twenty-four executions, and eight murders. Causes of death unfamiliar in modern times include the sixty-six who died of 'Evil', five who died from 'headmoldshot' (a disease affecting the sutures or bones of the skull), twenty-one died of lethargy, a surprising number, 410, died of 'Surfeit', and around five per cent of deaths were put down to problems with teeth.

Another interesting fact about life in early modernity was that some people had quite remarkable life spans. Statistics compiled in *Observations on the Past Growth and Present State of London* by Corbyn Morris in 1751, of burials in the City and suburbs of London, show that for 1740, the year this book ends, a third of deaths occurred in infants, so that first year of life was still a vital one, but also that a number of hardy people survived to their centenary and beyond.

Year	Total number of burials	Under 1	2-5	5-10	10-20	20-30	30-40	40-50	50-60	60-70	70-80	80-90	90-100	100+	Total number of christenings
1740	30811	10765	2862	1235	947	2205	2783	2866	2585	1977	1716	758	100	12	15231

***

As this introduction has set out, it is clear that the ways in which people interpret the body is governed by the culture in which they live. This is one of the reasons that historians of the body eschew any notion of retrospective diagnosis: if different elements or aspects of an illness are considered more important than others, then these are the ones a patient would describe and seek to have treated by their doctor. This means that some early modern diseases have no modern equivalent. This is not to do with ignorance; rather it is about rationalising the body within the familiar frameworks, which people knew to be 'true' of how the body works. Early modernity, as we have seen, was a time when ancient theories about the body were changing and being challenged, but it remained one in which the ancient truisms handed down from pre-Christian medical writers remained sovereign, meaning this book can span a 200 year period.

The sources for this book are as diverse as the illnesses it covers. Case notes kept by doctors and apothecaries are the obvious starting place and we have put these observations into the context of medical theories promoted in many published anatomy, disease, and medical treatises. As well as these, the book takes examples from personal correspondence, diaries, journals, and literature too. Handwritten books of recipes – known as receipts – still exist in some numbers and many are collected at the Wellcome Library in London. These contain the sorts of remedies that people made up at home at the time. The literate public also bought cheap almanacs listing the most auspicious days of the coming years along with significant religious days and local information, but these too often contained recipes for popular kitchen medical cures. Fascinating insights into our ancestors' relationships with their bodies can be found in court records too. Early anatomy guides were normally structured from the head down and while this is obviously not an anatomy guide, we will give a nod to the information we draw on from those books by ordering this book in the same way.

So, explanations and accounts of a range of common early modern maladies or complaints make up what follows. Some illnesses or conditions which were thought of as diseases in the past, we would now think of as symptoms of another disease; for example, jaundice might be taken as a symptom of liver conditions, but in many early modern treatises was written up and treated as a disease. In describing the way early modern people felt about the diseases they considered themselves to have contracted alongside an account of their diagnosis and treatment we gain a valuable insight into what it meant to be alive, thrive, and to survive in this era.

Part One

HEAD COMPLAINTS

Chapter 1

Migraine and Headache:
A Laborious and Dull Sense

My head is pounding. It feels like it'll break into twenty pieces
– William Shakespeare

On 26 January 1653, the Viscountess Anne Conway wrote to her good friend Henry More, discussing a book he had written and wearily recounting that she had 'been extremely troubled with a violent fit of the headache these 3 or 4 days'. Anne suffered terrible headaches throughout her adult life, which she considered to be a consequence of a fever when she was 12, and sought the help of some of the country's most eminent physicians including Royal physicians Theodore Turquet de Mayerne, and William Harvey, as well as Robert Boyle and Thomas Willis. At the time of writing this letter she explained that her headaches continued 'for all that Harvey hath hitherto done to me'.

Henry More thought that Lady Anne was partly to blame for her own suffering because she engaged extensively in study and intellectual endeavours, for which she was well known. He wrote to her in April 1653 to let her know that he had spoken to a new doctor, whom she wished to try on his recommendation, but noted that he thought Dr Ridsley would agree that:

> *you increase your disease by over much meditation. And for my own part I know it by experience, that intension of thoughts, and anxious considerations of things, will extremely heat a man's spirits, and call them up into the head. From whence it must needs follow, that those that are liable to the head-ache […] must needs increase that malady, by over much intending their brain.*

Lady Anne had apparently already countered this argument by telling More that she refrained from study and intellectual pursuits when she was feeling unwell. Yet her headaches continued.

As her string of physicians and second opinions suggests, Lady Anne tried a succession of remedies including opiates, tobacco, and mercurial treatments, which were nearly fatal. In 1656, forced by desperation and the severity of her pain, Lady Anne travelled to France to undergo trepanation. Again, sadly for her, this brought no relief. Just two years later her symptoms were so severe that both her relatives and her physicians thought she might not survive. Rather than lose her life though, it turned out that Anne was creating life – she was pregnant, although even this bodily change did not alter her sufferings.

In 1665 Lady Anne took a new approach. She made overtures to the healer Valentine Greatrakes, asking – through the Earl of Orrery – for him to come to her home, Ragley Hall in Warwickshire, to treat her. Greatrakes had gained renown for being able to cure people by touch alone. After the Restoration of the monarchy in 1660 he had 'discovered' that he had the power to cure the King's Evil (scrofula – see Chapter 16), a disease which had traditionally been cured by the thaumaturgic divine touch of the monarch – hence the name the King's Evil. In January 1665 Greatrakes was convinced to leave his native Ireland and travel to Ragley Hall. On his arrival he treated some of her tenants, his successes impressing both her husband and Henry More. Yet despite his fame and initial successes, Greatrakes repeatedly failed to cure Lady Anne's headaches. Her husband wrote to a friend 'Mr. Greatrakes hath been here a fortnight tomorrow, and my wife is not the better for him.'

In many ways Lady Anne was lucky, her privileged position and renown gave her access to a range of medical practitioners and headache medicines. But not everyone could afford such help, and for many a lie down was the best hope of getting through a headache. This had awful consequences for one 16-year-old Martha Gilbert. She told the Old Bailey in 1720 that she 'was much troubled with the Headache' on 30 September 1719 and so had gone to bed for a lie down 'about three or four in the afternoon'. While in bed, Thomas Belsenger went upstairs looking for the pot in order to relieve himself. On spying the teenager resting, he forced himself on her. This case was prosecuted at the central criminal court and several women spoke in Martha's case, but Belsenger successfully argued that the girl had flirted with him before, and with examinations of Martha's body leading to conflicting medical opinions by a midwife and a surgeon about what had transpired, he was acquitted. In the absence of effective treatments Martha had resorted to rest and relaxation in a bid to ease her head, leaving herself vulnerable.

Understanding Headaches

The surgeon and medical writer Philip Barrough explained in the *Practice of Physick* that there was a clear distinction between headaches and migraines. There were, he stated, three types of head pain described by Galen: inveterate headaches, or *Cephalea* in Latin, such as those suffered by Lady Anne, 'an old pain that hath long continued'; *Cephalalgia*, a head-ache, which was 'nothing else but a laborious and dull sense, and feeling newly begun in the whole head'; and *Hemicrania* or 'migrime'. He was careful to note that headaches, of all three kinds, applied to the skull and parts of the head covered in hair, rather than the face, but conceded that sometimes headaches affected the skull, sometimes inside the skull, and sometimes only half of the head.

Barrough explained that while different types of headache might have different causes, they were usually attributed to humoral disruption or an evil quality of the humours. An abundance of humours gathering in the head caused many headaches, or a blockage that stopped the passage of the humours away from the head and brain. Robert Johnson agreed that 'vapours, and humours, fuming up [from the stomach and other parts] to the Head' were the predominant cause of headaches. Headaches caused by excess heat or coldness were, he explained, more vehement, while those caused by dryness were more moderate. If these humours were of a biting quality, then the pains would be 'pricking and shooting'.

As today, headaches were also a known consequence of excessive liba-tions and drunkenness. Levinus Lemnius's treatise on the *Secret Miracles of Nature* explained to readers that drinking usually ended in either sleep or vomiting, but that in both scenarios 'the head will ache the next day'. Drink was thought to cause excess vapours that afflicted the head and the brain. On the 8 February 1660 Samuel Pepys recorded in his diary that having drunk 'a great deal' with his 'old friend Dick Scobell' he had come home to bed with his head aching.

What does appear to be absent from these descriptions of the causes of headaches is head trauma. But the wider populace did acknowledge that such accidents caused headaches. Poor Pepys noted on 21 July 1663 that his head was aching all day because he had knocked it 'against a low door in Mr Castle's house'. This added insult to injury as his head already ached as a result of a restless night's sleep. Yet others, like Yorkshire gentlewoman Alice Thornton, did not relate head traumas to headaches. She recorded in her autobiography that when she was just 3 years old she had been walking along holding her nurse's 'coats' (skirts) because her nurse was occupied with holding Alice's infant brother. Being unable to keep up, she wrote, I 'stumbled against the threshold & fell upon the corner stone of the hearth [...] At which time I broke the Skull of my forehead in the very top.'

The injury was serious enough for her to be in 'great danger of death, being like to have bleed to death', but Alice noted that her mother's careful ministrations and remedies allowed her to recover, with only a 'great Scar' to remind her of God's mercy at allowing her to live. Despite the severity of the injury Alice made no mention of any headaches that occurred as a result.

Hats for Headaches

As with most diseases, patients could attempt to cure headaches by rebalancing their humours. At least one writer argued that applying leeches to the temples (or haemorrhoids) to remove or draw excess blood away from the head could ease 'old and stubborn' pain. Herbals, and other botanical works, also described several plants that were thought to ease the pain and tension of headaches. Robert Lovell's 1659 herbal suggested that the juice of the plant houseleek eased headaches, as did chickweed drunk in mead. Another medical text suggested that the herb rue placed up the nostrils or sodden in wine and then eaten, eased headaches by clearing the brain and removing phlegm. Robert Johnson recommended a medicinal white wine, but only 'For the Rich', which contained elecampane, rue, sage, vervain, sweet marjoram, aniseed, sweet fennel seed, and orange peel.

A number of medical practitioners, usually unlicensed, also advertised cures through handbills. These single-sheet advertisements generally listed all of the ailments that a physician could cure, or advertised a particular medicine, normally a panacea that worked marvellous and wonderful effects in a range of disorders. One advert, possibly produced in the 1690s, offered the 'Grand Balsamin' pill for sale. This, the author assured readers, eradicated all '*Aches*, and *Twinging Pains*, and other *Distempers* of the *Head*'. Likewise, sellers of 'Saffold's pills' noted that they removed 'Pain in the Head' and the sellers of the '*Excellent Universal* PILL' claimed that it cured headaches. It was not always clear in the adverts what ingredients such pills and potions contained, but the effusive language and relative cheapness perhaps made these drugs an attractive option.

Many remedies suggested for headaches and migraines took the form of plasters and hats, which applied medicinal herbs and plants directly to the head. Some of these plasters were relatively simple mixtures of ingredients spread over linen and applied to the forehead. Elizabeth Okeover's handwritten recipe book, for example, suggested a plaster that was made as follows, 'take the juice of Betony & vinegar with crumbs of brown bread make it into a plaster & lay to the forehead as hot as it can be endured: pro:'. The final note here, 'pro', is an abbreviation for *probatum est*, the Latin phrase for 'it has been proved', which suggests that at some point this remedy was made, used, and was believed to have had a beneficial effect. Thomas Vicary's *Englishman's Treasure* (1641) included a similar remedy, except it recommended red mints and leavened wheat bread mixed with vinegar.

Recipes like this included a variety of ingredients. The book of Mary Chantrell (and others) claimed to have 'the best thing as ever was for a hot burning headache' – a 'pennyworth' of oil of pompilion (black poplar) rubbed into the temples and crown of the head with warm burdock leaves then placed on the top of the head and the temples. While Mrs Corlyon's book included a remedy made from a handful of wild daisies mixed with a 'dozen great earth worms' and an egg white, this was then spread upon a forehead-sized piece of linen, taking care that it reached the eyebrows and the temples. Alternatively, the book attributed to Sir Thomas Osborne advised taking ox gall with drag-on's blood (the gum or resin derived from the dragon tree), nutmeg and egg white, again applied to the forehead and temples as a plaster.

Lady Ayscough's recipe book dated to 1692 recommended a slightly more complex procedure, which produced a medicinal cap rather than a plaster:

> *For the Megrim or giddiness of the Head, Take Betty sweet marjo-ram rosemary of each one handful dry them to powder put to it white frankincense mastic cloves nutmegs cinnamon of each half a spoonful cast the powder upon the scarlet flocks carded quilt them in taffeta sarc* [a garment worn next to the skin like a chemise] *next make a cap & wear it.*

Johnson also suggested a quilted cap filled with the powder of sweet marjoram, vervain, betony, sage, chamomile flowers, nutmeg, cloves, aloes and galangal, amongst other ingredients. Before application the patient's head had to be shaved and the scalp rubbed gently to better open the pores. This created a more permeable bodily boundary for the healing ingredients to cross more easily to ensure efficacy.

For those who did not want to sit with a cap on their heads, or who had need of greater mobility (although who is to say these caps couldn't be worn outside) there were other options. John Locke noted of his travels in France that a man there made silver and iron rings, which people wore to ease their migraines. He claimed that 'He sells many and therefore [...] they may have some effect.' In Italy there were reports that one Giuseppe Rosaccio sold a ring made from bone, of hippopotamus tooth as it was claimed, which was good for headaches.

Prognosis

As headaches varied in their cause, intensity and duration there were difficulties for healers trying to offer a prognosis. However, one Hippocratic aphorism printed in a collection in 1610 claimed that 'Those which are in health being suddenly taken with headache and thereupon presently become dumb, and snort, do die within seven days, unless a fever come upon them in the meanwhile'. Robert Johnson repeated this same caution in 1684.

A shedding of watery matter or blood from the nostrils or eyes, Johnson said, signalled a sudden recovery. This was a 'crisis' point, looked for in most diseases as a sign that the party was overcoming the illness and so the patient was likely to survive. There was a caveat to this though, that if the pain was violent but suddenly vanished without this shedding of matter, recovery was very doubtful.

Headaches were also a sign that other diseases might be on their way. A headache accompanied by noise in the ears, deafness, or a numbness in the limbs could be a forewarning of apoplexy (a condition characterised by its suddenness and which robbed people of their sense and motion – akin to a palsy or a stroke), or an epileptic fit. A headache in someone prone to a choleric stomach might also be a sign of impending eye problems or foreshadow a loss of sight.

Like a Hole in the Head

One of the treatments Lady Anne Conway experimented with is perhaps one of the most famous medical treatments in the popular mind-set – trepanation. Drilling a hole in the head – using a trepan, or trepanning – is popularly assumed to have been undertaken to allow evil spirits to 'escape' through the head. But early modern surgeons were somewhat more pragmatic and used the operation principally in cases of skull fractures. It was not really then, according to medical manuals, of use in headache cases, but clearly some people, Lady Anne included, thought that it might bring some relief.

Drilling into the skull was, obviously, a serious operation. It was therefore important to identify whether it was really necessary. There is evidence that people tried to diagnose skull fractures at home, before seeking the help of a surgeon. The recipe book attributed to Johanna Saint John included a method 'To know a Fracture or whither the scull be broke'. This involved placing a knotted thread between the patient's teeth. The tester held the other end taught and then twanged, or 'twitch[ed]' the thread 'as you do the string of a viol when you try if it be in tune'. It was important to twitch the string very vigorously. If the patient could not endure two twitches of the string, but instead felt 'like a Dagger in his Head' then it was a sure sign that the skull was fractured. Corroborating signs were a pain when putting the teeth together or chewing meat, and a propensity to vomit.

The trepan was a round saw which cut the bone in a circular motion. They came in a range of sizes to make greater or smaller holes. The image that accompanied Ambroise Paré's description of these saws reveals that they were rather imposing, with a central pointed tip and a circle of sharp serrated teeth. An English translation of the French text *A Complete Body of Chirurgical Operations* (1699) explained that using a trepan allowed for splinters and shards of the skull bone to be removed from the brain, could facilitate the movement of depressed parts of the bone back into their original position, and made an opening that allowed medicines to be applied directly to the brain.

The operation was a dangerous one and medical writers discussed at length where on the skull it was safe to drill. One surgeon warned that the thick membrane surrounding the brain adhered very firmly to the coronal (the coronal suture runs across the top of the skull towards the front of the head) and the occipital bone (the bone at the back of the skull) and so these should never be drilled. Likewise readers were warned that the eyebrows were an unsuitable place for the trepan because the cavities beneath made the operation 'difficult and troublesome'. Establishing a safe place to trepan was only half the story though; surgeons were advised to think long and hard about whether it was best to proceed. Charles Gabriel Le Clerc advised that:

> *The Surgeon is to have recourse to his own conscientious Discretion, which ought to serve as a Guide, and requires that we should always act according to the known Rules of Art; insomuch that after having well considered the Accidents with all the Circumstances of the Wound, if there be no good grounds for undertaking the Operation, it is expedient to desist.*

Preferably a surgeon would seek the advice of a colleague rather than relying on his own judgement alone. Importantly for Le Clerc, this would protect the surgeon and keep them 'always secure from all manner of Blame', if something went wrong. Protection for the surgeon and patient was paramount because, as with all surgery, the stakes could be very high.

Sometimes though, the surgeon's choice was not the one that mattered. The surgeon Richard Wiseman recounted in one of his published observations how he treated a 10-year-old boy who had bruised his head falling from a horse. The accident stunned the boy who experienced vomiting and swelling. Wiseman made an incision into the boy's scalp to relieve the swelling. Given that the following morning the 'Patient [was] freed from the preceding Symptoms', Wiseman decided that the boy did not need more aggressive treatment. However, the boy's relations and friends thought that trepanning would 'prevent farther dispute', so Wiseman 'complied with them'. Not only did he agree to perform the surgery, he let the family choose the instrument he would use. Having examined a 'Trepan and Trephine' they 'unanimously preferred the Trepan'. Thankfully the boy recovered and Wiseman's surgical interventions were credited not only with healing this particular injury, but also removing a general susceptibility to headaches and vomiting that the boy had experienced since infancy.

Headaches ranged in severity from the minor inconvenience associated with a hangover, to the chronic problems of Lady Anne Conway, and even the pain associated with a fractured skull. The range of remedies was likewise diverse, from the standard efforts to rebalance the humours, such as by using soothing caps worn about the house, to serious and life-threatening operations, showing just how troublesome headaches in this period could be and how desperate the sufferers could become.

Chapter 2

Epilepsy: The Sacred Disease

'Did Caesar Swoon?'

– William Shakespeare

One of the many English translations bearing Nicholas Culpeper's name, this time of Felix Platter's *Golden Practice of Physick* (1664) described how 'every *Epilepsy* is horrible and abominable, which the ancients therefore called *the sacred Disease* as sent by the Gods by way of punishment, and others have Superstitiously imposed the Names of the Gods on it'. In addition to the sacred disease, Sir Thomas Eliot's 1538 Latin dictionary translated *epilepsia* as 'the falling sickness', and epilepticus as 'he that hath that disease'. This name probably arose because collapsing in convulsions is the best-known symptom of the disease. Most people knew the disease by this name, or sometimes as the 'falling evil', and although Henry Lyte used the term 'epilepsy' in his *New Herbal* in 1578, it did not become fully naturalised into English until into the seventeenth century. The origin of the formal term is the Greek 'to seize', which obviously then led to epileptic episodes being described as seizures.

While some ancients viewed epilepsy as having supernatural origins, this was not a view held by the author of the Hippocratic text *On the Sacred Disease* who instead explained that 'men regard its nature and cause as divine from ignorance and wonder, because it is not at all like to other diseases.' Roman historian Suetonius (70-130) offered another explanation for the name in his biography known as the *Twelve Caesars*, which was available in English translation from 1606. He explained that the sacred disease was so named because it affected the head, which was 'the most honourable place of the body and the seat of the Soul.' This text described how Julius Caesar suffered from epileptic seizures, a detail which William Shakespeare depicted in his 1599 play. In this play, Casca describes to Cassius and Brutus how Caesar 'fell down in the marketplace, and foamed at mouth, and was speechless' (1.2.250), to which Brutus replies that it is well-known that Caesar has 'the falling sickness'.

In biblical times some people argued that fits were the result of demonic possession, and this was a view that had some standing in the early modern period too. In 1667 Oxford physician Thomas Willis published his second groundbreaking book on the brain, *Pathologicae Cerebri*, following on from *Cerebri Anatome* (1664), which came complete with detailed illustrations by Sir Christopher Wren. Samuel Pordage translated Willis's work into English and it was posthumously published in 1684 with the snappy title *An Essay of the Pathology of the Brain and Nervous Stock in which Convulsive Diseases are Treated of Being the Work of Thomas Willis*. It explained 'many who were taken to be *Demoniacs*, or possessed with the Devil in the *New Testament*, were only Epilepticks; and that they called the cure of this Disease by our Saviour Jesus Christ, an ejection or exorcism of the evil spirit'. Echoing Hippocrates, Willis wrote that it was the fact that the disease was so hard to understand that caused it to be thought of as supernatural: 'In truth, in this Distemper, no marks at all of the Morbific [disease causing] matter appears, or are so very obscure, that we may have deservedly suspected it to be an inspiration of an evil spirit'. That said, like with most maladies, early modern people were more interested in a medical cure, combined with prayers for health, than they were in pursuing notions of possession. Although ideas of possession varied according to the religious denomination of a worshiper, an incident noted in the biography of non-conformist preacher Vavasor Powell, by Edward Bagshaw (1671) describes how Powell claimed to have cured a number of people including:

> *Elizabeth Morris of new Radnor, (a Religious Maid) having the Falling sickness or Convulsion Fits, which took her many times in one day, one night being at Family-Duty in a Brother's house in Town, whilst I was speaking she fell into one of her Fits, but Prayer being made for her she recovered before the prayer was ended, and for many years had no more fits, and I think hath not been troubled at all since.*

In this episode, prayer cured her illness; Powell didn't discuss possession.

Signs and Symptoms

On the Sacred Disease taught that epilepsy was a hereditary disease and that it was more prevalent in people with colder, wetter humoral balances, which was a hereditary trait too. Over-accumulation of phlegm was at the heart of the cause. The brain was conceptualised as a membrane holding fluids, which in turn absorbed and distributed air. If, as was the case in the phlegmatic, the person was congested, caused by the cold phlegm congealing on contact with warm blood, then the air could not flow in the veins and ultimately fits would happen.

It is common for people with epilepsy to get a warning of an impending episode, sometimes called an aura, and early modern texts noted this too. Polish physician Joannes Jonstonus's (anglicised to John Jonston) *The Idea of Practical Physick* (1657) – yet another translation ascribed to Nicholas Culpeper – listed the typical signs of an imminent epileptic fit:

> *the trembling and quivering (as it were) of the Nerves, splendours and bright shinings like unto the Rainbow flying and waving to and fro before the Eyes, the sense and smelling of some offensive stench, the Vertigo, and the yellowness of the Veins under the Tongue*

Jonston described the signs that a fit was taking place as:

> *a sudden falling, a Contortion (as they call it) or writhing of the Members of the Face, very improportionate unto, (or bearing no proportion withal) the matter thereof, a kind of Roaring and Howling noise that they make, the gutting, and close clashing together (or as they call it, Collision) of the Teeth, the shutting and fast holding together of the Fingers, an involuntary and insensible letting out of the Urine, and sending forth the other filth and Excrements, foaming and frothing like unto the white of an Egg, &c.*

The excess of phlegm was a ready explanation for why people would foam at the mouth during a fit. As Jonston explained, a 'thin or frothy' humour would accumulate in the brain and irritate the nerves 'and thereby introduce a constriction and straightening of the Passages' whilst at the same time the body would try and rid itself of 'what is noxious and offensive', this was what caused the loss of the senses and the convulsions to start. Fits were broken down into those that lasted for a long time '*diuturnal*', and shorter ones. Differences in severity were also categorised.

Willis proposed that a chemical reaction caused epileptic fits. He described how certain nitrates and sulphates in the blood gathered in the brain, and travelled in the same creeping motion as a worm, down the spinal column, in the vital spirits or spinal fluid, and into the blood and then the muscles. If these chemicals met in the muscle then 'by reason of instinct', or the action of the muscle, they would 'explode' and cause a spasm. Willis was aware that the term 'explode' was controversial, but his lengthy justification of the word shows that he meant something akin to 'reacts with'. Willis rejected the humoral phlegmatic idea as he claimed to have performed post-mortem examinations on many people who had the beginnings of their nervous system covered in 'limpid water' but who never suffered from the disease.

Childhood and Adolescence

Children were known to be susceptible to a form of epilepsy that they might outgrow. Convulsions can be common in very young children, especially when associated with a fever, but childcare manuals in early modernity warned of the dangers of startling or frightening babies as this could provoke epilepsy. The consequences of such seizures could be severe. In a poignant diary entry, dissenting minister and physician James Clegg described the death of one of his young children from convulsions. In March 1720 he noted that: 'My dear child Ebenezer was seized about the first day of this month with very strong convulsions which continued above a week and increased in violence till the poor babe was brought into a weak state.' Clegg recorded that he:

> tried many means to procure it ease and followed the use of them with earnest prayers for success – the fits left it for several days but on Sunday last it was, its lungs were clogged with phlegm and [I] apprehended the convulsions that had seized the internal muscles of the Thorax and in one of these fits the sweet creature expired in [my] arms on the Lord's day in the morning about six.

It is usual in the case of severe fits for the sufferer to be unable to swallow. Ebenezer Clegg was just a week short of his three-month birthday when he died on 13 March 1720, leaving his father distraught.

Therapies

Like Caesar, Shakespeare portrayed another protagonist as epileptic. When Othello collapses, Iago describes how 'My Lord is fallen into an Epilepsy. This is his second fit: he had one yesterday'. Cassio tells Iago to rub Othello's temples when he falls into a fit, but Iago thinks this would make him worse, saying instead that

> No, forbear.
> The lethargy must have his quiet course.
> If not, he foams at mouth; and by and by
> Breaks out to savage madness. (4.1.45)

Being left to recover in a quiet space is good advice when a fit is in progress. Philip Barrough endorsed Iago's view in his 1583 *Method of Physick*. Barrough's list of treatments to prevent fits is typically humoral, advising that the first thing a sufferer should do is amend their diet to include 'things that will attenuate, cut, and divide', or breakdown the phlegm. The room should be kept warm so that the air was hot and dry, especially if the patient was phlegmatic, which people with epilepsy were presumed to be. The sufferer was advised to:

> *eschew all flesh, except birds that fly on mountains: also he must avoid all kind of pulses, fish, & wine, especially if it be old and thick. Let his drink be* mulse [honey-based] *or thin ale: the eating of capers doth marvellously profit.*

Foods to be avoided included 'garlic, onions, mustard, & such like fumous things.' In addition, exercise was thought good, but Barrough cautioned against 'too much lechery' or sex, and 'let him sleep measurably on nights, and let him eschew exceeding sleeping on the day.'

As was seen in the case histories above, purging cures were popular both with the humoral and the chemical physicians. One case described in the notes of Lady Grace Mildmay concerned a 25-year-old Wiltshire woman who had suffered from epilepsy since childhood. Like the noblewomen healers mentioned in the Introduction, Mildmay had a reputation for making medicines to help out local people, and indeed bequeathed a bundle of medical notes to her daughter consisting of 'diverse books and more than 2,000 loose papers'. Mildmay decided that the best approach in this case was to make a purge and use sweating to expel the 'slime' that she assumed was blocking the young woman's uterine veins, so stopping her from menstruating, leading to an cachexy, or imbalance of humours, resulting in fits. This treatment lasted months but had the desired effect and the fits went away. Willis recommended regular vomits for his young patients alongside medicines such as peony, rue, mistletoe, and lily of the valley to close the pores in the nervous system. In the case of a fit, smelling salts made from oil of amber or hartshorn (shavings of the antlers or horns of a deer, or liquid ammonia made from this substance) intended to neutralise the explosions was his first choice. Some of these purges seem rather violent to modern eyes. John Locke's diary for 1678 included the suggestion that for chronic epilepsy:

> *the best method of curing is to shave off the hair, and use blistering ointments over all the head, so drawing the virulent humours to the*

surface; leave the little ulcers longer to infect the skin of the head, so that over a period of time those serous humours may seep out through the ulcers. I have even seen the most stubborn head disease cured in this fashion.

One of the more outlandish cures for epilepsy was menstrual blood. Roman historian Pliny, whose ideas were still being recited in this era, explained that menstrual blood had many startling properties, such as the ability to make a dog mad should he taste it, kill whole fields of crops, or to drive bees from their hives. It could also blunt knives, make iron go rusty, dull a mirror, and had the power to make an unwitting suitor fall in love if some of the woman's powdered blood was slipped into his drink. But this magical substance had good effects too; the 1651 translation of Henry Cornelius Agrippa's books of *Occult Philosophy*, borrowed from Pliny by repeating that 'it is said that the root of Peony being given with Castor, and smeared over with a menstruous cloth, cureth the falling sickness.' None of the more mainstream medical treatises seem to have taken up this advice however.

Before the Reformation people could access a range of objects that they trusted would aid healing. Catholics prayed to the saints and touched their relics in order to access divine power, and wore folded prayers on the body like charms. After the Reformation, the Protestant church frowned upon such activities and deemed them superstitious and irreligious. This did not, however, put a stop to such practices entirely, and throughout the early modern era medical texts made notes about the amulets and charms employed to cure diseases. William Salmon's *The Practice of Curing* (1681) recorded in a series of observations that for falling sickness, 'Amulets hung about the Neck, or born at the pit of the Stomach, are Counted useful; the fresh roots of Peony, cut into little squares, and being strung like Bracelets, and hung about the Neck, and as soon as they are dry, let new be put into their places.' He also explained that vervain (verbena), mistletoe, elks' hooves, and hypericum (St John's wort) worn in the same fashion might offer a patient some relief.

Obviously there was no way of definitively diagnosing epilepsy and ballads tell of roguish beggars feigning the condition to arouse sympathy. In a similar vein, Anne Miller claimed to have epilepsy when she appeared in the dock at the Old Bailey in London on 9 December 1691, where she was indicted for breaking into widow Anne Badger's house in Stepney. A man warming himself in front of the fire caught Miller red-handed, stealing household items including a waistcoat valued at ten shillings, but she claimed that 'she was troubled with the Falling Sickness, and so fell into the house, the door being open.' The judge dismissed this as a 'frivolous excuse' and found her guilty.

Despite new chemical theories like those of Thomas Willis set out in his treatise on nerves in the second half of the seventeenth century, it wasn't until the nineteenth century that the nature of epilepsy as we currently understand it was discovered. So while now we understand that it is a condition caused by an electrical imbalance in the brain, throughout the period covered in this book, epilepsy was largely seen as a humoral imbalance to be treated by diet and purging primarily, drying herbs in the long term, and sometimes opiate sedation in the case of an epileptic episode.

Chapter 3

Palsy: Paralysis or Shaking

'And with a palsy fumbling on his gorget, Shake in and out the rivet'
– William Shakespeare

On the 21 May 1691 John Evelyn received word that his nephew, who bore his name, had died. The younger man had been sick for some time and the physicians had despaired of his recovery. However, all of a 'sudden he began to mend'; his previously lost appetite returned and he became cheerful once again. He was, according to reports, well enough to venture out of his chambers and even out of the house. John senior recorded that sadly, this was his nephew's undoing, and that taking the air in his coach one day had caused a vein to break somewhere in his body. The young John perished because nothing could stop the blood loss caused by this turn of events. This might not have been a fatal event, but John noted that his nephew's existing bodily state was not robust enough to deal with the jolting of the carriage. He claimed in his diary that despite previously being 'strong & robust' and 'of very good sense', his nephew's drinking had weakened his constitution: 'so great was the sharpness of his blood, & [so] weak the vessels, which inconveniences accompanied with a Palsy, was contracted by an habit of drinking much wine & strong waters to comply with other young intemperate men.' Young John Evelyn thus died aged 35. Palsy was a key element in this young man's death, contributing to a weakened bodily state that could not cope with the rigours of disease and recovery.

Evelyn attributed his nephew's palsy to his excessive consumption of alcohol. But alcohol was not the only liquid capable of disrupting the body. One of John Hall's patients, as recorded in the 1679 edition of his observations, developed the condition because of her consumption of water. Mrs Wilson travelled to Bristol because she thought she was afflicted with the stone. While she was there she drank too greedily of the restorative waters of St Vincent's well – reportedly she drank eighteen pints a day. This caused a drastic cooling of her body and she fell into a palsy. To remedy this she moved once more, this time to Bath, where a combination of bathing and purging restored her health. In both of these cases palsy caused, or was a complication of, another disease. People seem to have experienced palsy as both a symptom, as a disease in its own right, and as part of ageing.

Palsy in early modern England could refer to two different bodily experiences: partial paralysis, or uncontrolled shaking. Some authors distinguished between the two kinds by referring to the former as a 'dead palsy'. More often than not it was this form of the condition discussed by medical writers. Further distinctions were made depending on how much of the body was affected. An eighteenth-century textbook based on the work of French physician Lazare Rivière explained that if it affected the whole body then it was a *Paraplegia*, and if it affected half of the body then it was called a *Hemiplegia*. It was a disease in its own right, but many diseases shifted, changed and mutated into palsy over time, as Mrs Wilson's story implies. John Locke noted more than once in his writings that colic and 'looseness' could both degenerate into palsy. Bridget Hyde's manuscript recipe collection from the late seventeenth century also suggested that this disorder was associated with apoplexy (or stroke). She labelled her remedy for the condition 'The great Palsy water for Apoplexies.'

The cause of palsy was an abundance of phlegm obstructing the nerves and thereby hindering the passage of what Galen had termed the *Animal Spirits*. Many authors, including Levinus Lemnius, explained that these spirits were the principal instruments of the soul and were responsible for the various actions of the body. The animal spirits were made in the brain and were responsible for motion and sensation – hence why their disruption led to loss of feeling and trembling. Excessive drinking, the consumption of narcotics, or the 'steam' given off by quicksilver, could all produce these offending humours. William Salmon, the empiric and medical writer, published a patient history, similar to Mrs Wilson's experience, in *Iatrica: Seu Praxis Medendi. The Practice of Curing* (1681). In which a young man 'too plentifully drinking Wine' fell into the disease. Salmon explained that he experienced 'Stupidity and Numbness' in his right hand, causing him to drop a glove he was holding. When the young man then attempted to get up out of his chair, his right leg wouldn't oblige and finally a 'kind of Heaviness and Unsensibleness' overcame him. What normally might be taken as signs of intoxication were in this case seen to be much more threatening. Tumours near the nerves could likewise cause an obstruction. Finally, cold, as Mrs Wilson discovered to her detriment, could prevent the brain from adequately distilling animal spirits. And as the revised version of Rivière's book explained 'Ice; the cold Air, a wet Cloak kept long about the Neck [...] sometimes to bring the Palsy.'

One question that occupied medical thinkers at this time was why some-one who experienced an injury on one side of their head (or body) would experience paralysis and palsy on the opposite side of their body. Helkiah Crooke writing in the early seventeenth century explained that most peo-ple agreed that this did happen, but that the cause was 'much disputed'. Some believed that the nerves of the body crossed each other and so, because they intersected, damage to one side of the body was transmitted across the body. A second school of thought argued that the nerves didn't intersect, but crossed from their point of origin to the other side of the body. Crooke dis-missed those who believed in the first model, because, as he claimed, it was obvious that only the optic nerves came together at any point. In all other cases the nerves were clearly defined and did not cross each other.

By 1721 when the nerves and the nervous system were becoming much more central to theories of disease, an anonymously authored med-ical treatise on disorders of the *Head, Brain and Nerves* could claim that 'a Resolution or Relaxation of the Nerves from their due Habit' caused palsy. This relaxation then caused a loss of motion and sense. This author described the disease as 'perfect' when all sense and motion was lost, and 'imperfect' when it was diminished causing 'a Trembling or Shaking of the Parts affected'. Things hadn't moved on too far though, because the author still noted that one of the causes of a relaxation of the nerves was an accu-mulation of cold humours.

Shaking Palsy, Witchcraft and Ageing

Although paralysis of the limbs could affect anyone and was associated with a range of other diseases, palsy characterised by shaking developed some particular associations with witchcraft. It was not always that the disease was caused by malefic means, but the language was useful for describing the symptoms. For example, in 1589, Robert Throckmorton's five daugh-ters were all bewitched. The family lived in Warboys, Huntingdonshire, and were attacked, supposedly, by local residents John and Alice Samuel and their daughter Agnes. Jane Throckmorton, who was only 10 years old at the time, suffered from a range of symptoms including bouts of loud sneezing that lasted for half an hour at a time, fainting and falling into a trance, swell-ing and 'Sometimes she would shake one leg and no other part of her, as if the palsy had been in it, sometimes the other: presently she would shake one of her arms, and then the other, and soon after her head, as if she had been infected with the running palsy.'

Initially Jane's mother believed her suffering was natural. When Alice Samuel visited the sick child and Jane called her a witch, the mother rebuked her and thought that Jane's weariness was triggering an over-active imagination. Jane's urine was sent to Dr Barrow for a diagnosis but he replied saying there was nothing wrong with her, although perhaps she might be troubled with the worms. After a series of purges and repeated analysis of various urine samples sent to Dr Barrow, he urged her parents to consider whether she was, in fact, bewitched. Robert and his wife held out against 'any such conceit of witchcraft' until, precisely one month after Jane had fallen sick, two more daughters were stuck down with the same symptoms and again 'cried out against Mother Samuel'. The confusion here between witchcraft and illness was not uncommon, as witches were thought to inflict illness and disease, along with other strange symptoms, on those who had crossed them. In many cases people turned to witchcraft as an explanation for ill health when doctors had failed to find a natural cause.

Although Jane and her sisters suffered from palsy-like symptoms in their youth, trembling was more commonly associated with the elderly and the gradual decline of their bodies. Lady Sarah Cowper kept a diary as she entered old age. In it she recorded with some disdain that an acquaintance 'Sir T.L.' had married a 'lady old, decrepit with the palsy and other infirmities.' As the woman was rich, Cowper concluded that his motivation, as many thought, was greed. For the most part Cowper was disgusted by the idea that this couple would engage in sexual activity, something that she thought was completely unacceptable for the elderly to do. However, to show the bodily state of this old lady she chose to emphasise the palsy, suggesting that, to her at least, it was a clear marker of ageing and infirmity. Unfortunately Lady Cowper was not to escape the condition herself. In the summer of 1716 she recorded in her diary, which had been her solace throughout her old age, that 'I feel myself decay apace. O Lord! give me grace to wait patiently till my change come'. Eventually, aged 72, she stopped writing in the diary altogether, explaining rather melodramatically in September of that year that:

> *The palsy increases on my hand so that I am forced to leave off my diary, writing is so troublesome to me –*
> *… My phrase now is farewell forever.*

An Obvious Condition

The author of the reissue of Rivière's book mentioned above was quick to say that 'The *Diagnosis* of this Distemper is easy': if the body was insensible to feeling or unable to move then it was obviously experiencing palsy. He claimed that finding the place of the obstruction or oppression of the nerves was also sometimes easy if it was the result of an injury. Internal causes, though, might be much more difficult to pin down. For these the physician should consider whether the patient was old, or favoured a cold and gross diet. It was important to identify the disorder swiftly because the limbs affected – cut off from the animal spirits and nutrition – would start to wither. Medical writers acknowledged that this was a tough disease to cure, in both children and in adults – but that didn't stop them trying.

Whips and Waters: Cures for Palsy

Some of the cures for this disease may appear extreme to modern readers. John Locke reported that chemical physician van Helmont had cured a young woman in Rotterdam who had lost the use of 'all her parts from the hips downwards'. He achieved this by 'ordering' the girl's mother to 'whip her soundly with rods'. As an aside, he noted that whipping with nettles might be even more beneficial. These methods were perhaps intended to stimulate the area of the body that had lost sensation. A more common approach was to use an infused water to treat the condition. Several family collections recorded recipes for palsy water. Mrs Carr's recipe collection included a version of the water made with borage, bugloss, cowslip flowers, sage, rosemary, and betony. These herbs and plants had to be collected as they came into season and added to spirit of wine. Separately, lavender was steeped in spirit of wine for twenty-four days in the sun, distilled, and the resultant extract added to the original mixture. To this already complex remedy were added: an ounce of balm, motherwort, bay leaves, spikenard leaves, orange flowers, six drams of citron pills dried (or lemon pills), hulled peony seeds, an ounce of cinnamon, nutmeg, cardamom, cubebs, yellow saunders, and finally, one dram of aloes. Johanna Saint John's palsy water was very similar and she directed that the patient should take forty drops of the water on sugar, or the crumbs of bread, at night when they were going to bed. She also recorded a recipe for a 'Palsy Balsam' attributed to Lady Barrington. This contained a different set of ingredients, including juniper berries, sarsaparilla, and castoreum (the secretion from a beaver's perineal glands). She instructed the maker to steep the ingredients along with lavender and rosemary flowers in brandy in the fireplace for four nights. To this was added camphor in spirit of wine. These remedies were very complex and required substantial investments of time, effort, ingredients and skill. But the remedy in Johanna's book at least suggested that such efforts were rewarded because the remedy would 'keep [for] 20 years'. If it was required, therefore, the process didn't have to be repeated on a regular basis.

The overall aim of these cures was to remove the obstruction by weakening the cold and thick humours clogging the nerves. But, as medical writers repeatedly stated, the disease was difficult to tackle and cures were not always successful. The drunken young man described by William Salmon was treated by a 'learned Physician' who recommended the full therapeutic range of phlebotomy, vomits, purges, cupping glasses, scarification, liniments, frictions and other administrations; metaphorically throwing the entire treatment book at him. None of these actions worked and his palsy 'still grew worse'. Although initially he had retained his mental faculties, after eight days of languishing he 'fell into a Delirium', experienced convulsions and died.

These examples show that while palsy was often seen as an affliction associated with age, it could in occur in anyone, and was even thought to be something a person could induce by intemperately drinking too much alcohol or water. While the causes were disputed, all agreed it was a tricky condition to treat and the outlook for sufferers wasn't great.

Chapter 4

Eye Complaints: Light without Heat

'It is most true, that eyes are formed to serve'
– Sir Philip Sidney

The 1587 English translation of French physician Jacques Guillemeau's *A Worthy Treatise of the Eyes* explained that of all the senses, sight was the 'most dear and precious' to men. This was because, unlike animals, men's heads and eyes were elevated towards God. Guillemeau praised the way in which the eyes, the most beautiful and 'most perfect' work of God, were given to man 'principally to see therewith and to guide and direct him to the knowledge of God, by the beholding of his fair and goodly works.' Works that no other sense, he believed, could adequately comprehend. Thus the eyes were intrinsic to faith, and so accorded a privileged place in the understanding of the body. Indeed in ancient times, philosophers like Plato supposed that vision worked by means of divine fire in the eye. This fire cast out light into the world enabling sight, but this notion was considered metaphorical rather than factual in early modernity. Still the loss of sight was both physically and spiritually distressing for early modern people. Some, like dissenting minister Isaac Archer, read sightlessness as a direct punishment from God. He recorded in a diary entry for April 1665 the story of a 'poor maid at Chippenham who had been vain and foolish enough, and now God had deprived her of the sight of both her eyes.' He rather piously went to visit her and encouraged her to consider how the 'blindness of her body might be for the enlightening of her mind', even though he admitted to himself that he wouldn't have the inner grace to accept this either.

On a more practical level, many people also relied upon their sight in order to earn a living. This is not to say that those who lost their sight were always unable to work. Margaret Pelling's study of the occupations of the urban poor found that ten blind, or almost blind, people appear in the Norwich census for 1571; of these, eight were unable to do anything to support themselves, but one continued to work as a baker, while an 80-year-old woman still knitted. Some people found ways to mitigate the effects of poor eye sight or compensate for it. A 12-year-old orphaned boy accompanied one blind man in his fifties acting as his guide. The author John Milton famously went blind in 1652, aged 43. The reason for his sudden loss of sight is not clear, but he was obliged to compose his epic poem *Paradise Lost* (pub. 1667) by dictation to various people, including his daughter. Milton published a touching sonnet in 1673 about the condition, *When I consider how my light is spent*, detailing how he had had to spend half his life in a dark world. Compensating in various ways gave people some measure of independence, but in all likelihood it was still a difficult life.

As with all aspects of health in the humoral system, a two-fold strategy was needed to ensure healthy eyes. First, people could avoid risking their eyes by adopting a good lifestyle and regimen; second, they could utilise a range of medicines to combat particular ocular afflictions. *Two Treatises Concerning the Preservation of Eyesight* published in 1616 and attributed to the sixteenth-century doctor Walter Baley, explained that if possible, people should avoid living in wet places, that 'Southern winds do hurt the sight', and that low dusty rooms and smoky places could all jeopardise eye health. Likewise he recommended that people eat easily digestible foods like hens, pheasants, and wild doves, which were 'greatly commended' for their ability to preserve ophthalmic health. He claimed that all writers agreed that doves eaten alongside turnips 'hath great faculty to do good to the eyes, and to preserve the sight'. On the other hand people should avoid all 'Gross and slimy meats'. Baley picked out small birds like martins, swallows and jays as especially dangerous – although he noted it was only the 'common people [who] happily may be compelled to eat them'. Baley was also disparaging of fish, but allowed that, prepared in certain ways, 'some fishes, which do scour in gravely-places' might be eaten without 'great harm'. Baley described in detail each of the groups of foods available to early modern men and women, outlining which salad herbs, fruits, nuts and drinks affected the sight.

For those who were particularly concerned about their sight Baley also recommended making and taking medicines designed to protect the eyes from ill-health. Eyebright (the herb euphrasia) 'and other things comfortable for the sight', he argued, could be made into medicinal drinks and taken with food in the morning if the patient could 'well endure' them. Other medical writers made similar suggestions. A book of Dr Lower's remedies from 1700 recommended his *'famous Water'*, made by distilling a loaf of rye bread, and administering it as eye drops. This book likewise recommended eye drops made from the water released by burning a Holland cloth (a type of dull linen) between two pewter dishes.

Two hundred and forty Diseases

There were many disorders that could afflict the eyes; Jacques Guillemeau claimed there were 'an hundred and thirteen', while the antiquary William Oldys claimed in 1753 that there were '*Two hundred and forty Diseases*', from swellings in the eyelids to cataracts. We can infer the range of conditions that people experienced from the range of remedies found in early modern remedy collections. Some were simply to soothe sore eyes. Sir Thomas Osborne recorded Mr Tukes's remedy, which contained wild woodbine and plantain leaves boiled in 'rain water gathered in June clear from the clouds', subsequently mixed with verdigris, alum and English honey. To use this mixture the patient added some rosewater and dropped it into the eye with a feather. Other manuscript recipe books were more specific and aimed to remove particular disorders. Remedies for 'pins' 'pearls' and 'webs' in the eyes were particularly common. These conditions caused obstructions to vision and might have been awkward when navigating daily chores and activities. One remedy for the pin or web in the eye, for example, required horehound mixed with honey and wine to be dripped into the eye.

As well as these homemade remedies, many people also sought the help of doctors and surgeons when they had eye problems. John Locke recorded in his diary that 'My Lady Banks had a swelling on the edge of her eye lid with swelling and redness of the veins in the inside as bloodshed. Dr Turbervill cured it with a decoction of red rose and damask rose leaves in barley water applied with a sponge.'

Spectacular Spectacles

Failing eyesight was a common feature of ageing in this era, as it is today. This process could start relatively early. Several diarists noted their despondency as their sight dimmed and expressed fears that they would lose their sight altogether. Lady Sarah Cowper recorded in her diary in 1709, at the age of 65, that her sight was failing her along with her intellectual capacities: 'Now I find thro' age, griefs, and infirmities, my sense is become dull, my memory decayed, my sight failing, my hearing imperfect, and in all the powers and faculties of my mind and body great debility.' Similarly in May 1669, after almost a decade of diary-keeping, Samuel Pepys reluctantly gave up the practice as his sight was simply too bad to continue:

> *And thus ends all that I doubt I shall ever be able to do with my own*
> *eyes in the keeping of my journal, I being not able to do it any longer,*

*having done now so long as to undo my eyes almost every time that I
take a pen in my hand [...] And so I betake myself to that course, which
is almost as much as to see myself go into my grave: for which, and
all the discomforts that will accompany my being blind, the good God
prepare me.*

For some, spectacles could compensate and correct failing eyesight. Pepys
himself trialled a new invention, consisting of cardboard tubes 3 inches
long which acted like binoculars. On 11 August 1668 he recorded being
'mightily pleased with a little trial I have made of the use of a Tubespectacall
[sic] of paper, tried with my right eye'. He took this to work with him and,
on 28 August, noted being able to read a letter without pain, to his great
joy. Known of in Europe in medieval times, spectacles were only made in
England from the seventeenth century, and although still very costly, were
common enough for William Shakespeare to use in Jacques's famous 'Seven
Ages of Man' speech from *As You Like It* in which 'The sixth age shifts
to the lean and slippered pantaloon / With spectacles on nose and pouch
on side' (2.7). George Willdey and Timothy Brandreth advertised their
'Incomparable Spectacles and Reading-Glasses' in the *Daily Courant* in
1707, emphasising their skill as artisans by warning potential customers that
'false Common Spectacles draw and damage the Eyes'. Unlike these dubious and potentially risky glasses, Willdey and Brandreth boasted that their
lenses were eminently beneficial: 'By the use of these Young Persons may
preserve their Sight to old Age, and the weakest Sight so assisted as to be
capable of Reading the smallest Print or doing the finest Work.'

By 1724 it was even possible to buy specially prepared glasses that allowed
the wearer to safely view an eclipse. These were likely to have been more
common than the strange glasses offered for sale in the 25 April 1676 edition
of *Poor Robins Intelligence*:

*These are to give notice that Peter Pinchbelly Baker, dwelling in Light-
loaf-Lane, intends, at the next Sessions to sell his share in a pair of
Spectacles, which are made of substantial two inch Board, not to be
worn upon the Nose, but the Neck and Wrists, through which a man
may clearly see his faults, and his Enemies, and he made feelingly sensible of the swift flight of Goslings, Ducklings, and Chickens, while they
remain in the cloister of the Egg-shell; they are fit for all ages, from
Eighteen to Threescore, and teach such as use them, the most difficult
distinction between good and evil.*

Eyes Made by Art

In addition to spectacles, some early modern oculists also offered false eyes for clients who had lost an eye to disease. Such a purchase was limited to the wealthy, who could afford to spend money on an item that did not have a practical benefit. Samuel Hartlib, an educational reformer and writer from Poland who spent most of his adult life in England, was certainly aware of the possibility of buying such items and noted the following advert in his ephemerides (diary) for February – May 1650:

> *Any Gentleman or others that hath lost an Eye by any Casualty whatsoever, may have an Eye made by Art (to take away that great blemish) so Exactly that it shall not be distinguished from the natural. By John Thomas dwelling in Campions Lane, Thames Street, near Allhallows the Great.*

One Richard Herring owned a glass eye, listed as part of the haul stolen from him on 16 July 1721 by John Storey, along with a pair of boots, three razors, a cloth waistcoat, and a pair of breeches. Herring valued his possessions at forty shillings but, although Storey was found guilty of the theft at his trial at the Old Bailey the following month, the jury determined that the goods had a value of just ten pence, meaning Storey could be transported for his crime rather than hanged, as the true value of the goods would dictate. Since Herring was presumably not wearing his glass eye at the time of the theft, it means there is no way of knowing why he owned it or if it was something he wore regularly.

Couching for Cataracts

Although many eye difficulties were treated with drops, washes and waters, cataracts posed a more serious problem. The name comes from the similar Latin term, *cataracta*, which means a barrier like a portcullis or window grate, since the cataract veils the vision like these physical barriers do. Randle Cotgrave's 1611 French–English dictionary has an entry for '*coulisse:* a portcullis [...] also a web in the eye'. This was a very common condition and one avenue of treatment was to have the cataracts removed. Surgeons and other, sometimes less reputable, specialists performed couching for cataracts. There was some discussion about how this operation was discovered with some commentators offering interesting explanations. The surgical treatise of Daniel Le Clerc from 1699 claimed that curing cataracts in this fashion had been discovered 'by observing that *Goats*, that were troubled with 'em, recovered their sight by having pricked their Eyes with rushes, or thorns, as they brushed through the Woods.'

Despite goats supposedly being able to perform the procedure, surgery was not always an easy option. Like all early modern surgery, couching was not to be undertaken lightly. Presumed to be caused by a phlegmatic humour, the build-up of superfluous humours between the cornea and crystalline humour, as Dutch surgeon Paul Barbette explained, could be either imperfect – where the eye was not totally covered – or perfect where the material covered the eye and had transformed into a membrane. If the humour was still soft, still admitted light into the eye, and could be moved with a needle, the operation could be undertaken. Those who could no longer see the glimmering of light when they looked into the sun were thought to be past help. The patient would be sat in a chair with his eye bound and covered and the surgeon sat opposite in a higher chair; the patient was asked to 'clap his hand about your waist, without stirring them at all as long as you are busy in the Operation.' An assistant held the patient's head from behind, while the surgeon held the eyelids open, and the patient looked down towards his nose. The surgeon would then 'quickly thrust [the] Needle into the *Cornea*, half a straws breadth from the *Iris*, and bring it unto the hollow of the Eye; when the Needle hath touched the Cataract, endeavour therewith to press it gently, and so long from above downwards until it remains there', once this had been achieved, the needle was withdrawn and the eye bound with linen, rosewater and egg to heal.

Stories circulated of successful cataract removals. John Dury (also Durie) the preacher and ecumenist wrote to Samuel Hartlib in 1654 referring to the eye problems of a mutual friend, probably the same John Milton discussed above as Hartlib and he were acquainted (Milton dedicated his 1644 pamphlet on educational reform to Hartlib, claiming to have written it at his friend's urging). His letter makes clear that cataracts and sight loss caused despair and sadness, but that people had faith that surgical intervention could remedy the problem. He wrote:

> *I wish that Mr Milton may recover his sight; & I would not have him to despair of it; because I was told that an old man of threescore & odd years who had been 10 years blind in the territory of Schaphusen* [in Germany] *was cured by an oculist a husbandman in those parts who took a Cataract from his eyes which had covered them so long time, & now he sees perfectly again.*

The age and inveterate nature of this man's condition should have made the cure quite difficult. Milton himself denied that he had cataracts and wrote that his eyes were 'externally uninjured. They shine with an unclouded light, just like the eyes of one whose vision is perfect', so this treatment wouldn't have been suitable for him. However, even more extraordinary cases were published to underline that couching could restore lost eyesight. William Oldys published the case of William Taylor of Ightham, Kent, treated by London based John Taylor. William had apparently been born with cataracts in both eyes. John convinced him to undergo the operation when he was 8 years old. Although William was reluctant, John explained to him that if left alone 'he would be deprived of all Ways to get his Livelihood; must be a Beggar-boy, in want of Clothes and Victuals', moving from door to door and having nothing to depend on. Convinced by these arguments, William endured the operation and showed great fortitude in controlling his body and keeping his hands in his pockets so that he didn't have to be tied down; William's cataracts were swiftly couched. Indeed, after operating on the first eye, William reported with 'a Kind of wild Transport, and Wonder' the 'strange Shapes, Forms, and Colours of many Things, so incomprehensible about him.'

The ability to restore sight in cases like this raised interesting questions for oculists of this era. In particular William Molyneux, John Locke and others began to question whether those who had been blind their whole lives but who had their sight restored, would be able to identify objects from sight alone. They wondered whether these patients would be able to recognise something they had only previously felt and had described to them. Following the restoration of William's sight it was noted that he had difficulty gauging distances and had to put his head very close to a table in order to pick up some coins laid out on it.

Chapter 5

Toothache: Rotten Worms

'there was never yet philosopher that could endure the toothache patiently'
– William Shakespeare

Any time spent in front of the television today is enough to know that a clean, white smile is an important social indicator in modern society. A bright smile reveals a lot about the effort a person puts into their appearance and can reveal a lot about health as well, as stains and blackening can be caused by smoking, drinking or excessive caffeine consumption. Popular depictions of past dental hygiene, or a lack of it, tend to exaggerate to provide a sense of distance. However, caring for the teeth and gums was an important part of early modern health regimes. Medical texts warned of a variety of disorders and diseases that could afflict the mouth, while drugs and 'dentifrices' were offered for sale and made up in the home to help whiten the teeth.

David Perronet, a surgeon, sold his *'Salt of Cloves'* priced at just 6 pence that 'wonderfully cleanseth and whitens the Teeth, and preserves them and the Gums from Putrefaction and Decay'. 'Dentifrices' (preparations of either powder or liquid for cleansing the teeth) like this one date back to ancient times. For example, Philemon Holland's 1601 translation of Roman historian Pliny's first century works noted that the best ingredient in a dentifrice was ground pumice. In the eighteenth century these were widely available commercially. Ruspini's dentifrice, powder and tincture, was accompanied with instructions to place a 'sufficient quantity' on a brush and then brush both the teeth and gums on the inside and outside very well, rinsing with a sponge dipped in warm water. Households also recorded similar recipes for keeping the teeth clean and white. A collection of recipes attributed to Robert Boyle included *'A good and innocent Dentifrice'* made of mastic and dragon's blood – the plant resin rather than the blood of dragons of legend. In addition, most people used toothpicks to clean debris from their teeth. Higher-ranking people often owned ornate ones, and famously Henry VIII gave Anne Boleyn a small gold one as a courting gift in a set that also included an ear-scoop for removing excess wax.

Despite these good intentions early modern men and women suffered from a range of oral health problems. The works of Lazare Rivière, a seventeenth-century French doctor and professor at Montpellier University, were co-translated from Latin into English by Nicolas Culpeper in 1655. This text reveals that black and rotten teeth, erosions of the gums, bleeding gums, and mouth ulcers were all problems faced at this time. Toothache was perhaps the most common and inconvenient of these problems. Pepys recorded on 8 May 1661 that his wife Elizabeth had had a sore tooth extracted, or 'drawn' as it was usually called, that day. He then explained on 7 June that she was much troubled with a toothache. For Elizabeth, it appears, this was not an issue that was easily resolved. In December 1663 Pepys again recorded: 'My wife having strange fits of the toothache, sometimes on this, and by and by on that side of her tooth, which is not common.' Elizabeth had this tooth extracted on 28 December which left her 'pretty well'. However, she continued to suffer various bouts of toothache and on 18 December 1667, Pepys again recorded that she was 'exceeding ill in her face with the toothache, and now her face has become mightily swelled that I am mightily troubled for it.' Despite his concern about his wife, Pepys could be a little flippant about the suffering of others. In April 1663 he noted that his wife had taken a friend or relative named Ashwell to La Roche's to have her tooth drawn, but that she wouldn't suffer it after the 'first twitch'. He commented that this 'made my wife and me good sport' of the incident. On another occasion Pepys recorded his annoyance that Mr Rolt spoilt an evening of dancing and supper because his toothache made him poor company.

Pepys was not the only one to record the pain and discomfort of toothache in his diary. Samuel Jeake, a merchant of Rye in Sussex, noted on several occasions his experience of the condition. In some cases Jeake focused on the duration of the illness. For example, in June 1671 he noted that 'I was seized with a violent fit of the Toothache, which lasted 3 hours.' In June 1678 he experienced a particularly lengthy bout: 'A fit of the Toothache, continuing without intermission for 24 hours but not very violent.' As suggested here, the other defining characteristic of Jeake's experiences was the severity of the pain. In July of the same year he recorded that he was 'Troubled with the pain of the Teeth, which continued, but moderate'. Likewise, he recorded a 'violent pain in my Teeth all day' in January 1677. It is clear that like Elizabeth Pepys, Jeake suffered recurrent bouts over several years. Yet unlike Elizabeth, it is unclear whether he ever had his troublesome teeth removed. Either way it is clear that this was a persistent, uncomfortable and often painful condition to live with.

Numerous remedies for toothache circulated in the seventeenth and eighteenth centuries, intended either to remove the root cause of the problem or act as an analgesic. A sixteenth-century translation of *The Secrets of Alexis of Piemont* recommended boiling frogs in vinegar to create a mouthwash that was 'profitable for the pain of the teeth.' Jane Jackson's recipe book suggested a mixture of honey, bruised pepper, and the white of an oyster shell, melted together until it was thick and made into little pellets that could be put into the tooth, but didn't state whether this was to remove the cause or not. She simply described it as for the toothache. Elizabeth Jacob's book advised, rather counter intuitively, snorting up the nostril (on the side of the nose that corresponded to the pain in the mouth) a powder made from ginger, liquorish, and pellitory of Spain. Remedies to ease the pain of toothache could also be laid to the neck, the temples, and the ears. John Locke recorded in his journal that while travelling in France he met Mademoiselle Verchard. She had suffered from toothache for several years until she had had 'both her ears punched and kept from healing up again, with roots of Thymilaea [flax-leaved daphne]' which had greatly benefited her. Occasionally, he noted, the roots would cause an inflammation at which time Verchard would remove them and replace them with new roots that had been soaked in water and then dried. Some people also made use of rudimentary fillings: 'if a Hollow tooth draw it, or stop it with a little white wax.'

Like with most diseases at this time, not having the requisite materials to make a remedy in the home was not necessarily a hindrance to receiving relief from toothache. The proceedings of the Old Bailey, which were pamphlets detailing trials from the criminal court published regularly from 1674, carried advertisements for toothache cures. One from January 1707 described an 'infallible Cure for the Toothache' that not only relieved the pain but ensured that it 'will never return', a bold claim to make if Elizabeth Pepys and Samuel Jeake are to be believed.

Medical practitioners believed that toothache could actually be a pain of the nerves in the root of the tooth, the membranes around the tooth, or the substance of the tooth itself. This pain could have a variety of causes including a 'Flux of Humours'; either: cold and phlegmy, hot and watery, or salt and sharp. But they also believed that worms gnawing the insides of the teeth caused toothache. Evidence for the belief in tooth worms has been found in Egypt c. 1200-1100 BCE and in Assyrian medical texts, so it was not unique to this era. The *Practice of Physick* (1655) explained to seventeenth-century readers that 'there are also Worms in rotten Teeth, and they breed of any matter which is contained and putrefied in the Cavities, whether it be excrementitious [sic], or come of putrefying meats, especially flesh and sweet meats, which by reason of their clamminess stick to the cavities of the Teeth.' One method of easing toothache was thus to lure out the worms. One early eighteenth-century medical text named the worms as 'dentari' and explained that they

> *are commonly bred under a Crust that covers the Surface of the Teeth when they're disordered. These Worms are very small, having a round Head marked with a black point, the other Part of their Body being long and slender like those in Vinegar [...] These Worms corrode the Teeth by Degrees, and occasion a stink, but no violent Pains, for 'tis a mistake that vehement Tooth-Aches are occasioned by Worms.*

John Gerard, curator of the College of Physicians' physick garden, explained in his *General History of Plants* (1633) that the root of henbane was used by 'Mountebank Tooth-drawers which run about the country' to draw out the worms from people's teeth. They would, according to Gerard, burn the root in a chafing dish with coals while the patient held their mouth open over the fumes. He also claimed that particularly dubious practitioners would smuggle small pieces of lute string into the dish convincing their patient that 'those small creeping beasts came out of his mouth.'

When aristocrat Lady Elizabeth Delaval remembered having a bout of toothache as a girl, which had 'so many days and nights bitterly tormented me', she accepted that worms were the cause, and she recounted how:

> *My Head, my Eye, my Teeth, and my Neck are most miserably tormented with raging pain: All which a poor unlearned woman (with God's blessing) promises me ease of, she tells me that what I suffer is caused by the gnawing of little worms, that run along with the Blood in my Veins. I know, tell this now to any Learned Doctor of Physick and he will rather Smile at my simplicity, for expecting it to be Eased by this woman's skill, than not believe her more likely than to cheat than cure me.*

As the daughter of an earl it is reasonable to assume that she would have had ready access to a trained physician, unlike most people, but she took care to point out that the specific pain she was in would not have responded to any of their cures. She pitched herself as bravely going against the advice of those around her, and consulting an itinerant woman who, like others, might offer dental treatment as part of a range of health care options. Lady Elizabeth was ultimately vindicated when the unconventional treatment worked:

> *Most strangely has this woman surprised me, and many more here present. For behold here is no less than 200 Worms in this Basin which she has taken out of my Gums where (though I was willing to try her skill) I did not believe there had been any. But though I wonder much to see a plain Demonstration of what very few will believe, yet at the same time I consider we are far from Understanding all the secrets of nature; nor can I give credit to any man's judgment before my own eyes. Nor because this woman's Art [skill] in taking these little creatures of my gums (where they have so many days and nights bitterly tormented me) is unusual, must I therefore conclude it impossible to be done but either by witchcraft or cozenage.*

The scenario depicted by Lady Elizabeth, in which the woman took a quill and used it to draw lots of worms from her gums, is typical of the way this procedure was described in contemporary literature – when the assumption was that the quill was preloaded with the strings Gerard described.

Lady Elizabeth was alert to such methods, perhaps from reading the herbals or similar accounts and was quick to refute the possibility of this having happened in her case:

> *Most convincing arguments there are to me this woman deserves not the hated name of a witch, which many people give her, amongst the giddy multitude, whilst the mere sober sort reckon her to be a cheat; and that she cannot be neither, for 'tis impossible she can have been cunning enough (as has been reported) to put worms into my mouth through the quill with which she takes them out.*
>
> *I am sure she neither brought the quill with her, nor did so much as make it, for it was made by one of my own servants, and I plainly enough (as well as others) saw the worms stir (after she left me) in the water where she washed the quill that she opened my gums withal.*
>
> *Nay more, some curious people that were here took some of those little worms out of the water to try if they had life, and when they were cut in pieces we saw blood, which was a certain proof that they were not little pieces of lute-string which some incredulous people used to say she might slip into my Mouth with the quill with which she opened my Gums, and so washing it in the Basin she might make those pieces of strings move*

in the water, as if there were life in them; but these arguments were not made use of by any of those Persons who were Eye witnesses of the sudden cure that was wrought upon me.

She concluded that 'In fine, after all critical Arguments I dare affirm it for a truth that worms have caused those torturing pains my God has punished me withal and in his good time mercifully removed.' Lady Elizabeth's account appears in her spiritual diary and so she was keen to give God the credit for both the pain and the providential appearance of the woman healer.

Breeding Teeth

A common cause of toothache in children was, of course, teething, which was often colloquially called 'breeding' teeth. This is not now classed as a disease, but it was described as such in the past. The author of one treatise was careful to point out (probably to increase sales of his remedy) that the bills of mortality published in London showed that over '12000 Children yearly died of their TEETH, and Fevers, Fits & Convulsions caused thereby'. It is unclear from the bills whether they were actually talking of teething, or of tooth related problems in the wider population, as sometimes they only recorded the cause of death as 'teeth'. Indeed in a bill for August 1665, when the plague was raging in London, there were still 113 deaths credited to 'teeth'.

One popular method for curing this form of toothache was the wearing of an anodyne necklace. There were long traditions of making medicinal necklaces to hang around children's necks. Writing in the 1720s, John Quincy said that women made such necklaces out of peony roots. Numerous adverts for anodyne necklaces form part of a collection of seventeenth-century London handbills held at the British Library. One early eighteenth-century commentary on the necklaces claimed that, in combination with a liquid to soften and open the gums, they would ease the breeding and cutting of teeth in young children. The author even boasted that 'it's safe and easy Use, excellent Properties & Successful Effects' made it 'inferior to few Methods for Children in these Circumstances.'

Pulling or Falling Out

If toothache became particularly severe, as in the case of Elizabeth Pepys, then the tooth could be removed or 'drawn'. Rivière claimed that removing a 'very hollow' painful tooth would mean that 'the pain will presently cease and never return'. But he cautioned that if the tooth was drawn at the wrong moment, the brain might be damaged or the jaw broken, which could lead to a flux of blood, fever, and then death.

The pulling of teeth was generally the preserve of barber surgeons and specialist tooth-drawers, although there was increasingly a distinction that these men were inferior to true surgeons, despite the presence of some in the united company of barber surgeons. It was not until the later eighteenth century that dentistry began to emerge as a specialism with any considerable standing. Surgeons and barber surgeons had particular tools for this purpose, notably a pair of forceps used specifically to extract teeth.

Of course teeth also fell out, and it was relatively normal in early modern Europe for those of a certain age to be toothless. Jacques, in Shakespeare's *As You Like It*, famously alluded to this in his 'Seven Ages of Man' speech in which the final stage of life is a second childhood that left the person: 'Sans teeth, sans eyes, sans taste, sans everything' (2.7). Loss of the teeth was a clear sign of ageing and affected beauty as well as the ability to communicate and to eat. Those with disposable income could remedy the situation. Dublin surgeon Charles Allen's 1687 book *Curious Observations in that Difficult part of Chirurgery Relating to the Teeth,* devoted a whole chapter to the '*Restoration of the Teeth*'. Here he claimed that 'we are not yet to despair, and esteem ourselves *toothless* for all the rest of our life', as the 'loss indeed is great, but not irreparable'. Instead, he advocated filling a despairing hollow mouth with artificial teeth, which not only aided pronunciation but helped to preserve any teeth that remained and were 'a great ornament'. It was not only surgeons who performed such cosmetic work. One Mrs Norridge, lodging close to the Strand, advertised that she was 'very expert in cleansing the Teeth, and taketh out any perished part bewixt the Teeth; and cureth the Toothache, and the Scurvy in the Gums, and setteth in Artificial Teeth'; although the wording here is ambiguous about who produced those false teeth.

Artificial teeth were not the only option. Allen also explained that there was a 'Natural' process where 'rotten *Teeth* or stumps' were taken out 'putting in their places some sound ones, drawn immediately after out of some poor body's head'. He was, he claimed, less keen on this option though, because it was inhumane and was 'only robbing of *Peter* to pay *Paul*'. Better to use the teeth of dogs and sheep instead of human teeth as it was 'lawful', 'profitable' and 'advantageous'.

Part Two

ABDOMINAL MALADIES

Chapter 6

Disorderly Bowels: Griping Guts

'There's Emptiness, and Fulness; Flux, and Waste'
– Thomas Heywood

Reading through health guides, journals and diaries it is clear that early modern people were extremely attentive to their bowels. People often noted when they opened their bowels and what happened. They believed that medication, food and drink, weather and general health, all affected this function. As was discussed in the Introduction, evacuation was one of Galen's 'non-naturals' and so was taken seriously in monitoring health. In the humoral bodily economy, evacuations were an important means of balancing the body and maintaining health. Whereas we would describe going to the toilet and various synonyms for this, early moderns talked about going outside to the house of office, or easement, the privy, or the jakes. Inside the house, the wealthier would have a close-stool – basically a potty in an often ornate lidded box with a padded seat, sometimes with armrests. Most families used a pot of some sort inside at night and might have access to a communal jakes to empty them into. These were manually emptied periodically by 'night-soil' men; such a well-paid job that they were ironically nicknamed 'gold-finders'. Otherwise waste piled up in dunghills, which were the source of much litigation and bad feelings, especially in towns and cities. Social rank clearly had a bearing on people's toileting practices then. Chapter 18 contains descriptions of women who tried to dispose of babies in these communal houses of easement. The most polite term for excrement was 'stool' but 'shit' or 'turd' were in common parlance without the vulgarity these words tend to connote nowadays.

Since most cures sought to keep the body in balance, medicines to purge the body were widely used to combat a range of complaints. Lady Margaret Hoby noted in her diary that on several occasions she took a 'glister' or enema. These could be liquids injected into the rectum or a suppository tablet. Lady Margaret took one in 1599 after her prayers and spent a sociable evening. The treatment can't have worked satisfactorily as she repeated it the next day, which perhaps worked too well as she was forced to stay in her chamber until the afternoon. It was normal for doctors to note down the efficacy of these laxative treatments. A typical entry would be as in the case of Sir Thomas Puckering, who saw John Hall for vertigo, headaches and other symptoms. Hall determined that Puckering had a phlegmatic constitution and checked his urine, which he found to be 'well coloured'. Hall concluded that Puckering's symptoms revealed a digestive disorder, so he needed to 'empty' his patient in order to reset this. He prescribed purgative medicines taken at bedtime, which caused Puckering to have 'three stools in the morning'. More medicines were then taken in the mornings 'fasting' (on an empty stomach) and were 'divided into two equal parts; the first dose gave four stools, the other seven'. To maintain the improvement, Sir Thomas was given 'the foresaid prescribed Pills, three at night, and two in the morning, which gave five stools' and was apparently 'perfectly cured'. Similarly, Sir Simon Clark consulted Hall for a tertian fever, headaches and stomach ache. Hall again gave him a purge designed to expel excesses, and so the fever, from his body; this resulted in five vomits and eight stools. Taking these purges with some soothing hartshorn, this patient 'became very well' after three days of ministration.

'Obstructions in my Bowels': Constipation

As well as being considered a good idea to purge the digestive system in the case of numerous diseases, it was well known that constipation and its associated complaint of tenesmus was a condition in its own right. A posthumous translation in 1527 of German chemical physician and surgeon Hieronymus von Brunschwig's *The Virtuous Book of Distillation of the Waters*, explained that a pain in the guts known as tenesmus was when 'a man thinketh that he would go to stool, but he can do nothing.' Mrs Wincol, a 48-year-old chambermaid in the household of the Countess of Northampton, consulted John Hall for tenesmus where the straining had caused a 'falling out of the fundament', probably a rectal prolapse, or possibly a large haemorrhoid. Hall manually returned the protrusion to its proper place by heating the anus with hot linen cloths soaked in camomile and then using a finger to return the passage, holding it in place with a sponge. He noted that this delivered a perfect cure.

Constipation, or costiveness as it was more often known in early modernity, could be associated, like nowadays, with the more elderly patient as the digestive system became more sluggish with age. Chronic constipation can be a miserable as well as dangerous condition, as the ageing John Evelyn recorded in his diary on 1 May 1702: 'Not having the benefit of natural evacuation for several days, I was very ill, & feverish, but by God's mercy relieved, I began to be more at Ease, so I was able to go to Church this Afternoon [3 May]'. This episode turned out to be an uncomfortable but relatively light bought of costiveness, but he later recorded a much more severe incident. In March 1704 he claimed:

> *The beginning of this month I was so Indisposed with Obstructions in my bowels, not having the benefit of Evacuation for several days, that in my life I never suffered more torment, till after some Remedies it was removed & I restored again for which God be Eternally praised So as after a Week I was allowed to take the air.*

Evelyn didn't describe the remedies he took, but perhaps they were similar to those with which John Hall treated the 69-year-old Lady Katherine Hunks when she was 'cruelly vexed' with a high temperature, pain in her side and stomach, and also 'with a binding of the Belly for eight days'. Hall considered that she was in 'great danger of death' and so prescribed a clyster or liquid enema, which caused an immediate result of two stools. He treated her side with ointment and covered it with a buttered double thickness linen cloth. The clyster recipe was 'injected' again the next day, which resulted in three more stools. Hall's treatments worked, and along with a moistening diet, including currants taken on a stick of liquorice, and a barley drink, Lady Hunks was cured within fourteen days, for which he gave thanks to God.

'A Preternatural Disposition in Children'

Constipation can be very common in children caused by a lack of high-fibre foods, not drinking enough, or by problems with potty training or anxiety. Today's recommendations suggest that children should release their bowels three times a week in order to be considered healthy and normal. But the book of *Children's Diseases* by J.S. published in 1664 was rather adamant that 'Filth ought every day to be expelled'. The author claimed that costiveness was a 'preternatural disposition in Children' caused by an obstruction, a problem with the nerves and muscles, or by a weakness in the expulsive faculty. Importantly he explained that choler needed to be sent to the guts because it was this that 'stimulated and excited [the body] to an Expulsion'. Another cause of the condition was the production of thick humours that attached excrement to the guts preventing its timely release.

J.S.'s prognosis was rather severe, he claimed that it was a 'dangerous' condition in children because they were 'great eaters'. It was therefore vital to promote adequate bowel movements. To do this, medical books encouraged whoever was breastfeeding the child to eat '*Mallows, Dry Figs, Raisins*, and the Broth of *Coleworts*' (a type of brassica) and any other food that could 'loosen the Belly'. This was because medical theory dictated that the woman's milk would take on the qualities of the food she ate – food once consumed was converted into blood, which was then further changed or 'concocted' into other bodily fluids such as breast milk in women and sperm in men.

As in adults, there were various suggestions for medicines designed to stimulate excretion. J.S. proposed a suppository 'made out of hard Honey or the roots of *Mallows*; *Garlic* roasted in Ashes, and put into the fundament of the child'. An alternative was candied coriander, which he said 'tickles the expulsive faculty and causes no pain.'

Griping of the Guts: Diarrhoea

The opposite of constipation, diarrhoea (the suffix *hoea* always refers to a flow), was a term used by early modern medical writers, but people usually referred to this as a flux or a looseness. As the medical text of Michael Ettmüller, professor at Leipzig University, declared 'Sometimes it comes alone, at other times 'tis the Symptom of some other Diseases'. It was therefore like several of the conditions considered in this book, in that it could be a disease in its own right or a symptom of something else. In part, this ambiguity related to the humoral model, which focused less on specific diseases, than on what changes in the body revealed about underlying humoral complexion. Treating many conditions therefore focused on ameliorating symptoms rather than 'removing' a particular disease from the body. In particular Ettmüller linked looseness with *Phthisic* (a lung condition) and malignant fevers, but he also noted that some 'Cacochymical [ill-humoured] Persons' were liable to suffer a period of looseness that returned every quarter, year or month. Sharp, irritating humours that aggravated the guts or fermented the natural acid of the blood creating a mass of serum, operated like an induced flux from a purge.

Treating a condition that was characterised by the loss of bodily products or fluids posed an interesting dilemma for early modern physicians, as the go to measures of bleedings and purgatives were unlikely to help. *The London Practice of Physick* (1685) based on the work of Thomas Willis, and brought out by his own amanuensis and apothecary, Mr Flemings, mentioned that this was the case. It stated that there were two main types of flux, one accompanied by '*Griping of the Guts*' and one accompanied by bleeding. He claimed that in 1670, around the time of the autumn equinox, 'a World of People' fell sick with a dangerous flux and 'cruel Vomiting', which caused fainting and a total decay of strength. 'For the Cure of this Disease no Evacuation did good, nay Bleeding, Vomiting, and Purging always did hurt', rather it was important to use cordials of the hottest nature that abounded with spirit and sulphur to restore the body. He believed that brandy burnt with a little sugar was a 'Popular, and as it were Epidemic Remedy'. This remedy was evidently very successful, although the text cautioned against its use if the flow was bloody.

Warming and restorative drinks also featured in domestic remedy collections. An anonymous seventeenth-century book suggested that the patient take as much boiled milk 'as his stomach will bear once in 3 or 4 hours'. The patient was not to eat or drink anything else, but to keep warm and to have some embers from the fire placed under the 'stool' when they made use of it. Similarly, the recipe collection of Elizabeth Godfrey instructed two spoonfuls of rice to be boiled in three pints of water with a stick of cinnamon, and a handful of red rose leaves. Once the mixture had evaporated, conserve of red rose was added and the mixture was boiled for a little while longer before being strained and given to the patient.

Chapter 7

Jaundice: Shedding Choler

'The tawny Jaundice in her Eyes was spread'
— *Joseph Beaumont*

'The Jaundice is nothing else but a shedding either of yellow choler, or of melancholy all over the body' according to English physician Philip Barrough in the 1583 edition of his *Method of Physick*. The cause of this problematic shedding was a corruption of the blood, usually without a fever, which made it choleric. This was perhaps not too far off the mark since jaundice is caused by a build-up of bilirubin (a waste product created when red blood cells break down) in the blood. In this era jaundice was not always considered a disease in its own right, and although medical writers included chapters about it in their works, it could be a symptom that appeared in numerous other diseases. Despite not necessarily being understood as a disease in all instances, the Bills of Mortality did list patients who had died from the condition. In the bill detailing deaths occurring between 6 and 13 June 1665, only one person succumbed to jaundice. This increased slightly between 15 and 22 August 1665, the bill for which noted that three people had died from it. This was more than had died from gout, ulcers, kidney stones, or pleurisy, but it was still a very small figure. The number was rarely above four or five deaths a week.

Barrough suggested that jaundice, a term that borrows from French ('jaune' being the French word for yellow), also called *Icterus* in Latin, might be caused by an inflammation of the liver or a stoppage of the gallbladder either by a collection of matter or by a gallstone, a view modern medicine would support. Barrough and later, Robert Johnston, both also suggested that it was caused by the 'biting of venomous beasts', particularly vipers. Barrough proved this by recounting that 'a certain man, when he was stung of a viper, had all his body spotted like the colour of leaks.' Johnston similarly claimed that 'the external cause is the biting of a viper, whose poison is of a subtle, volatile, and spirituous nature; which doth soon render Choler over spirituous, after the biting of the Serpent.'

In early modernity, like today, medical writers and the wider populace knew that alcohol-induced liver damage could cause the condition. Johnston stated that:

> *Ebriety, or the abuse of strong drink, may be a procuring cause of this Disease, because the volatile spirit of the drink may be too plenteously mixed with Choler, which renders it spirituous, by which it becomes less apt to effervesce with the acid juice of the Pancreas, and hence most entirely to join itself with the other humours.*

If this was the case, he argued, sobriety was the key to recovery. John Hall treated a 28-year-old employee of his son-in-law Thomas Nash for the yellow jaundice, which was 'very much all over his Body'. The servant worked at the Bear, a tavern in Stratford, but Hall didn't mention whether excessive drinking caused his condition. The patient took an emetic mixture which produced 'seven vomits' and a laxative which 'gave him eight stools for four mornings', successfully curing him. Another of Hall's patients, however, definitely had drink-related yellow jaundice according to the case notes. Mr Fortescue of Cookhill Priory saw Hall in March 1633. He was 38 and 'a great Drinker, of a very good habit of Body, sanguine, very fat'. Fortescue had a myriad of symptoms including breathlessness, a hard tumour in his 'Belly, Cods [scrotum] and Feet'. Like Nash's servant, Fortescue had a purge, which produced eight stools, and also had blood let. Instead of beer to slake his thirst, he drank a liquorice and saffron infusion. Such was the severity of his condition that it took Hall a good six weeks and various combinations of treatment to effect a cure. Perhaps Fortescue's liver disease was more pronounced than Hall knew however, as historian Joan Lane has found that he died later that year.

Examining Excrement

Like several of the diseases covered in this book, diagnosis was considered to be rather straightforward. 'A Yellow Colour throughout the whole *Body*, more especially in the White of the Eyes' was the primary signifier of the disease. Accompanying symptoms included the tongue seeming bitter, hiccups, 'laziness' and itching. Elizabeth I suffered from jaundice in her youth, alongside digestive problems, anxiety attacks, headaches, and irregular menstruation. When a bout of jaundice overcame her in 1556, it was accompanied by difficulties breathing, which some took to be a symptom of the disease.

While these signs may have indicated the presence of the disease, they were not enough to pinpoint the cause of the condition. Thus Barrough argued it was crucial to 'consider the figure of the excrement, and the colour, seeing in some they appear much coloured by yellow choler, as also in some the urine doeth appear.' Looking closely at the body's waste products would clarify the state of the disease. He claimed that those whose choler had 'burst out unto the skin' because of a 'crisis' in a fever would have 'natural' coloured excrements. Alternatively problems caused by melancholy being sent to the skin and the blood would result in 'black urine, but their dung is like the colour the coperouse [sic] or shoemaker's bleach'. Finally, jaundice caused by an excess of yellow choler caused 'white egestions, their urines be coloured like saffron'. Careful consideration of these bodily by-products would, therefore, allow physicians to treat the patient's specific underlying humoral disruption or cachexy, not just their symptoms.

The Black Jaundice

In addition to the more familiar 'yellow' jaundice, early modern medical books also described '*The black Jaundice*' which was '*a change of the skin of the whole body into black*'. This illness was thought to arise from exactly the same causes as its yellow counterpart, except that rather than affecting the liver, these problems affected the spleen. It was distinguished not only by its colour, but by the fact that, as a translation of Joannes Jonstonus's *Idea of Practical Physick* (1657) declared, the 'humour is more stubborn' and there was a great 'fear of a dropsy' developing. The same text recommended 'Medicines of *steel*' (iron supplements) and dry baths to help ease the condition. Gervase Markham's instructions to *The English Housewife* (1625) offered suggestions for treating both conditions. For black jaundice he recommended the juice of pennyroyal or pennyroyal boiled in white wine. The recipe book attributed to Lady Ayscough evidently didn't follow this advice and instead recommended the following remedy for the black jaundice:

> *Take A pint of Earth worms such as creep out of* [the] *Earth after rain and put* [them] *in A dish & Strew A good handful of Basil upon* [them] *and cover very close when they have lain there one hour wash very clean* [with] *fair water* [then] *take* [them] *out of* [the] *Dish and beat very small & boil in A quart of White wine till they be almost half wasted drink of this every morning and every night for A week make fresh every 2 Days.*

'By Little and Little Departs'

Jaundice is a rather common and often harmless condition in newborn babies, known now as neonatal jaundice. The condition usually appears two or three days after birth and is generally gone by the time the baby is two-weeks old. The reason for its common occurrence is that babies' livers are yet to fully develop and so aren't as effective at removing bilirubin from the blood, and that babies have high levels of red blood cells in their blood which are frequently broken down and replaced creating bilirubin.

Some early modern doctors were similarly aware that the condition often appeared in newborns and would likely clear up on its own. Franciscus de le Boe, Latinised to Franciscus Sylvius, was born in Germany to an affluent family; as a physician he wrote a treatise on the disease of children, an English edition of which was produced in 1682. This book opened with a discussion of jaundice, explaining that it 'often appears in Infants soon after their birth, and continues for some days, and again by little and little departs'. He believed it was possible for infants to have the condition while still in the womb – evidenced by the fact that some children were born with a yellow tinge to their skin. Yet the authors of midwifery guides, which usually included a section on the diseases likely to affect newborn babies, did not very often include the disease in their works. Nicholas Culpeper, Jane Sharp, and François Mauriceau's book *The Diseases of Women with Child, and in Childbed*, all fail to associate the condition with infants.

Despite acknowledging that the disease often left of its own accord, Sylvius proceeded to offer a lengthy discussion on the causes of the condition in children and noted several cures. In particular he argued that oily and fat things, and those that procured sleep or stupefied the body were excellent cures: '*common Soap* dissolved in warm milk' was just one of his suggestions, because '*Soap* cures the Jaundice, First, *By its fixed lee Salt* … [and] Secondly, *By its thick*, not volatile and Aromatic *Fatness and Oil.*' Soap was made from fat, and Joseph Miller repeated this advice in the context of curing adults in 1722. Like all other authors he also recommended saffron, as well as opium: '*one Grain of Saffron* alone given them in their Mother's, their Nurses, or Cow's *Milk*, once or twice a day, often cures them of the *Jaundice*'. He concluded by helpfully noting that several of the medicines recommended for adults would do just as well for the cure of infants.

Saffron, Barberry, Dung, and Soap

The cures recommended for adult sufferers of Jaundice, like many seen throughout this book, could be rather unappealing to modern readers.

William Sermon's book *A Friend to the Sick* (1673) started with some rather palatable suggestions, rhubarb mixed with saffron and an electuary of the juice of roses, made into a bolus with fine sugar. However, the author then moved on to suggest dried and blackened egg shells beaten to a powder and given in white wine with saffron, or rooks' livers powdered and drunk in wine. Alternatively the 'fresh dung of a Goose that eats Grass in the Spring time' dried or the white part of Hen's dung made into a powder, were thought to be efficacious. Likewise sheep's dung mixed with the bark of a barberry tree infused in ale and white wine was proposed as a remedy. Joseph Miller's 1722 *Botanicum Officinale* claimed, as noted above, that,

> *Soap of any sort, conduceth to the cure of the Jaundice, upon a twofold account, both by reason of its fixt lixivial* [relating to Lye also used to mean alkaline] *Salt, and also by reason of its fatness or oil; for the Lixivial Salt doth correct and diminish the over volatileness and spiri-tuousness of the vitiated Choler, and the oil doth blunt the sharpness of the volatile and spirituous Salt ruling in Choler.*

Not all remedies for jaundice had to be consumed, and *A Friend to the Sick* recommended cutting open a live trout or tench, and laying it to the stomach as 'an infallible Remedy against the Jaundice.'

Saffron and barberry featured in many remedies for the jaundice because of their yellow colour. In a world where God had supplied cures for all ills, many believed that physical appearance was a clue to what a plant's curative properties might be, following the principle of like-follows-like. But herbalists and botanists claimed, without reference to its colour, that saffron opened obstructions of the liver, making it a well-known cure for the distemper. National pride was also apparently involved in advocating this cure. Joseph Miller was clear on this point, writing 'The best Saffron in the World grows in *England*, being cultivated in *Essex*, *Suffolk*, and *Cambridgeshire*'.

The meticulous and time-consuming work required to harvest the stamens from crocus flowers to produce saffron has not changed over the centuries. And so it was then, as it is now, one of the most expensive spices. In this way we can get a sense of the wealth and status of the families who kept collections of medical remedies, as they followed the convention of using saffron to treat jaundice. The manuscript collection of Sir Thomas Osborne included a remedy 'for the yellow Jaundices' composed of sixteen long knotted earthworms (collected in the evening) sliced and seethed in ale mixed with cloves and saffron. A second remedy in the book, which he attributed to Mr Sevill of Mexborough, combined saffron with the bark of a barberry tree and the tops of red nettles, the powder of hartshorn, and ivory. Lady Ayscough's book also included several remedies that included this costly component. The first recipe provided the following instructions:

> *Take eight Kentish pippins* [apples] *cut* [the] *Cores clean out then take 3 penny worth of Saffron & dry it then take 11 Sows for a man 13 if they be small for A woman 9 if they be small 11 bruise them with the point of A Knife altogether, then mix the Apple the Core being clean out with* [the] *Sows & Saffron put them into* [the] *Apple, coat it therewith eat one apple so ordered every morning for 3 mornings together then Omit 3 mornings & take it 3 mornings Again.*

Another remedy combined saffron with another strongly coloured spice: turmeric. These were beaten together to form a powder. Each morning and evening the patient had to consume as much of this powder as would lie on a groat, incorporated into a conserve of barberries or the 'pape' of an apple. She recorded a further two remedies for the yellow jaundice, one of which contained saffron, and a remedy that was designed to treat both the yellow and the black jaundice.

One of Lady Ayscough's remedies was 'For the Jaundice in case a woman lies in'. Jaundice in pregnancy is now relatively rare but can have serious implications for both mother and baby. It is not always caused by the pregnancy itself but can be the result of pre-eclampsia or *hyperemesis gravidarum*. In this case, Lady Ayscough recommended powder of dodder (cuscuta, a genus of yellow, orange and red parasitic plants) mixed with ivory, given in a syrup of lemons. While saffron may not have appeared in this particular remedy it evidently still relied upon plants that were yellow in colour.

Scarborough Spa

Given the rather unappealing composition of some of these remedies, we might expect that people looked for alternatives. William Simpson's book *An Historical Account of the Wonderful Cures wrought by Scarbrough Spa* may have offered just this. Simpson explained that 'it is found by observation [...] that those Medicines which do open obstructions are most prevalent in the cure [of jaundice], amongst which, those who abound most with a fixed or volatile *alkalie*, or partake of apperial Mineral Salts, are most effectual'. The waters at Scarborough were luckily 'fraught' with these laxative salts and so, taken alongside other remedies, were an 'adequate' remedy for the disease. As we have seen in several chapters of this book, the country's spas were popular healing destinations.

Simpson provided testimonies of several locals who used the spas for precisely this purpose. Sir John Legards' wife was perfectly cured by the spa in just a few days, for a jaundice that had 'long resisted remedies in a rational method'. Local minister Mr W. Hodgson also benefitted from the healing waters after six years of 'falling into the *Jaundices*, especially Spring and Fall'. For some it was the very localness of the spa that was important. The final case produced by Simpson emphasised that moving about the country could lead to ill health and that returning home for a cure was the best thing to do. He claimed:

> *Mr.* Palar *of* Nun-Noutain [Nun Monkton] *in* Yorkshire, *was during his abode in the Southern parts much afflicted with the* Jaundices, *having the symptoms which usually attend that Disease, consulted Doctor* Dickenson *(who then lived at* Oxford *but is now an eminent Physician in* London*) whose advice was to get him down into his own country and to drink the waters of* Scarbrough, *which he judged the best and most certain cure for him; whither accordingly he applied himself and in not many days was perfectly cured.*

Jaundice was a rather varied experience in this era. Sometimes it was a serious disease in its own right, and at other times it didn't have to be cured. Several medical texts explained that it might occur at the *crisis* point of another illness, as Barrough's diagnostic tests suggested. This was when the illness 'broke' either releasing its hold on the body and signalling the start of recovery, or signalling that a disease was liable to be fatal. Or in children, it might dissipate without intervention. Although we can't know, this might well have been a relief given that rather unappetising excremental nature of some of the remedies.

Chapter 8

Kidney and Bladder Stones: Easing the Passage

'A Man of My Kidney – think of that!'
– William Shakespeare

On the 26 March 1662, Samuel Pepys recorded in his diary with much joy that it was the four-year anniversary of his undergoing the 'cutting for the stone.' He wrote that he was in 'very good health' and 'like to do well.' Indeed he was, and despite occasionally complaining of pain when he caught a cold, Pepys remained free of the dreaded stone until three years before his death. Unfortunately, at this point, as Pepys wrote to his nephew Jackson the wound of this operation after 'more than 40 years perfect cure' had reopened. After his death, a post-mortem found seven stones in Pepys' left kidney weighing four and a half ounces.

Pepys was not alone, numerous men and women in early modernity, like now, suffered with kidney or bladder stones. The build-up of these small stones could be a relatively pain-free affair if they remained small enough to pass through the genitourinary system. However, many patients noted that large stones, or stones that were sharp and angular, caused considerable pain. Medical texts frequently used language such as 'great pain', 'torture', and 'much tormented' to describe the experience of the disease. Likewise, letters from the era convey a sense of the discomfort endured by those poor souls afflicted with the stone. Some long-standing sufferers wrote about their condition with familiarity, but did not downplay the severity of the pain they experienced. Sir Francis Harris wrote to Lady Joan Barrington on 4 September 1629 that he had not been well, and at that very moment was 'crazy of my old pain, the gravel, and fits of the stone'. The chronic and extreme pain induced by the condition became in itself a condition worthy of treatment in some medical texts. William Salmon offered remedies in his medical treatise for convulsions brought on by the pain of the stone.

Physicians believed that an excessive build-up of corrupt humours within the urine caused kidney and bladder stones. In hot bodies these humours 'baked' or hardened into troublesome stones that would obstruct urination or tear the bladder causing bleeding and pain. As discussed in the Introduction, younger bodies were humorally hotter than older bodies. This meant there was a contradiction evident to medical writers that old men were more likely to develop the disease than younger ones. The explanation for this was that old men had a weak 'expulsive faculty', which meant that they did not expel their urine with as much force and vigour as younger men, so the matter with the potential to become a stone spent more time in the kidneys, where it hardened into a stone. Because heat was a factor in the creation of kidney stones, eating 'hot' foods (all foods, like humans, were thought to have a humoral balance and quality) could provoke the disease. The medical works of Lazare Rivière, claimed that foods including beef, pork, hare, goose, shell fish, cheese, milk, hard eggs, chestnuts, pears, quinces, medlars (an apple-like fruit), unleavened bread, and anything produced by smoking, was a danger. Similarly, foods that were diuretic and moved matter to the kidneys too quickly might trigger the condition. A person's lifestyle also posed a risk: those too given to down beds, baths, sexual activity and lechery, violent exercise, anger, and other great passions, were thought to be prone to the disease. These were also personality traits and activities associated with heat. In addition to this, several medical writers discussed a 'stone-making spirit' that was particularly strong in some people's bodies and meant they produced larger, and more, stones than others. As mentioned in the Introduction, women's looser, wetter, bodies were assumed to be less prone to this condition.

'A Sharp Pricking Pain': Diagnosing the Stone

The presence of a kidney stone was indicated by several symptoms, including heavy dull pain around the loins, disrupted urination, or blood in the urine. When a stone moved into the ureters, a 'sharp pricking' pain supplanted this dull pain. An 'itching in the Yard [penis], which makes the Patient scratch it often', revealed a stone in the bladder, according to Rivière. But to be certain, physicians and surgeons inserted a catheter into the urethra to try to locate the troublesome concretions. Needless to say, some patients found the prospect of this examination most unappealing. A physician writing to Sir Hans Sloane, the Physician-extraordinary to Queen Anne from 1712, noted that a Mr Coteworth, one of his patients, 'has a great prejudice to being search[ed] for the stone and so much that I believe he will never submit to it.' The surgical treatise of Paul Barbette also noted that 'this searching was so very painful, that it was difficult, through fear of pain, to have it permitted a second time'. Thus he claimed that surgeons had to become better adept at identifying stones without an internal examination.

Even without surgical intervention, bladder and kidney stones were, at least, very uncomfortable to pass. At worst they posed several dangers. They could cause a stoppage of urine, resulting in tearing and inflammation to the genitourinary tract, which could lead to ulcers and fevers. Medical writers lamented that if the disease was hereditary, or the proneness to it was hereditary, then it was incurable. In old men it was also thought to be very difficult to cure. Although this might make us think that children were safe from these problems, Rivière commented that children's greater expulsive faculty meant they were less likely to get kidney stones, but more likely to get bladder stones, as any stones that formed were quickly pushed into the bladder. He continued to say that these stones remained in the bladder longer because children were often asleep or at play and so urinated less frequently. Moreover, their passages were still narrow and small, meaning the stones couldn't naturally pass out of the body, increasing the likelihood of surgery being necessary. In a diary entry for 3 May, 1650, John Evelyn, while on his European travels, documented how:

> At the hospital of La Charité I saw the operation of cutting for the stone. A child of eight or nine years old underwent the operation with most extraordinary patience, and expressing great joy when he saw the stone was drawn.

Reflecting on the experience Evelyn said that: 'The use I made of it was, to give Almighty God hearty thanks that I had not been subject to this deplorable infirmity.'

Showing off the Stones

Despite the discomfort associated with this disorder, or perhaps because of it, physical specimens of bladder stones appear to have given men bragging rights. The surgeon Matthew Purmann explained in his early eighteenth-century medical treatise that a Lieutenant Colonel of the Hannover Troops had, in 1687, shown him 'a great Box full of Angular, Oval and Round Stones' that he had voided by urination over a six week period, the largest of which 'was about the bigness of a great Pea.' Similarly, George Thompson, a chemical physician, added an appendix to his book *Galeno-pale: A Chymical Trial of the Galenists* (1665) in which he related the story of Anne Taylor. Thompson included a drawing of Anne's stones and welcomed visitors to his home to examine them for themselves, claiming that his friends had insisted he do so because they were so 'prodigious and monstrous'. Displaying things expelled from the urinary tract was perhaps not as unusual to early modern men and women as it might seem to us. In another instance, Staffordshire physician Richard Wilkes noted in his diary for 1739 that a Mr Smallwood of Lichfield showed him a 'Parcel of Worms, which he had voided by Urine; about a Dozen.'

Radishes and Cranberries as Cures

All sorts of remedies were recommended for easing the passing of stones and to prevent their build up. Some aimed to lubricate and soften the passages allowing them to pass out of the body with greater ease. Others claimed to break up the stones inside the body, again facilitating their natural expulsion. Finally, some remedies aimed to halt the growth of existing stones and prevent new stones from forming. Samuel Hartlib was at the centre of an extensive letter-writing network. He was known for sharing knowledge and books, and was associated with the printing of at least sixty-five pamphlets on a range of topics from religion to chemistry. In 1642, and then in his forties, Samuel began to suffer from the stone; by 1656 his condition confined him to his house. Many of his friends and correspondents wrote to him about his problems and actively sought remedies that would alleviate his suffering. While it is clear that his friends knew of his suffering, some of them weren't clear about the specifics of his disorder. Lady Ranelagh wrote to him that she had found a French surgeon in Dublin who claimed to possess a good cure and would be happy to help Hartlib if he would confirm that his stones were in his kidneys. A later letter from 1661, though, included a remedy for stones in the bladder. It might in fact have been, as medical writers emphasised, that it was hard to know the details of the problem because stones moved from the kidneys into the bladder, and from there into the urethra, in each of which location they could cause distinct problems.

Hartlib's friends could be rather ingenious in sourcing remedies for him. John Winthrop, colonial governor and physician, had John Richards ship a barrel of 'the best cranberries' and 'a barrel of Indian corn' from Boston to London, as he believed that the corn was 'easy of digestion & very diuretic & it hath been observed that whiles people used most of that food it was rare to hear of any troubled with the stone.' Not all remedies were so exotic. Samuel recorded in his personal papers that 'A knight in Cheshire with many others have found a wonderful deal of good in the stone by using the powder once a week of dried Haw's drunk in white wine.' Medical sources, including *Choice and Experimented Receipts in Physick and Chirurgery* (1675), also recommended hawthorn powder. Despite Hartlib's continual search for a remedy, his letters suggest that he never found adequate relief from his condition.

Many remedies for the stone used radish as a key ingredient. Indeed, some rather bizarre stories circulated in the medical literature to explain how such a common ingredient was discovered to have such coveted medicinal properties. *The Poorman's Plaster-box* (1634), for example, included the following lengthy story, which suggested that, in addition to showing off their stones to friends as discussed above, men also made cutlery out of kidney and bladder stones:

> *A certain High Dutchman, being very well skilled in cutting for the Stone, was on a time called to an old Gentleman, which was very much troubled with that Infirmity, he having searched him, found the stone to be of such an extraordinary bigness, that he would not deal with it, a while after this Gentleman died, he being acquainted with his friends, desired to open him for to see the stone, in brief he did, and found it so great, and of such a length, and hardness, that he wondered thereat, for it was so big that he made a haft for a knife thereof; this knife he being once at supper left on the Table, and the cloth being taken up, the knife was (unwittingly) taken up with it, and so cast on one side with the fragments; next day he missed his knife, and search was made for it, and it was found in a voider* [rubbish bin], *amongst scraping and pieces of Radish roots: but so strangely altered that he greatly wondered thereat, for through the virtue of the Radish (against that disease) the haft was found wholly to be consumed: which made him ever after, for to use Radish, against that disease.*

The author concluded that he would not deign to state whether the story was true or not, but did recommend radish roots steeped in white wine as a cure for the stone.

John Hall noted treating a young widow, one Mrs Winter who was 'troubled with the Flux of the Belly, Inflammation of the Reins, with great abundance of Urine, even almost to fainting; she was also troubled with the Stone and Scurvy confirmed, and was much weakened.' For this multitude of symptoms, Hall drew up a prescription for an electuary containing powdered hartshorn, coral, and bezoars. Hartshorn was a mild sedative, and taking just a drop of this mixture bound in poppy corn syrup, such as would fit on the end of a knife, Hall declared Mrs Winter much better. He also prescribed some laxative medicines and more hartshorn in a drink, which, he declared, cured her in just a few days. John Locke also treated a female patient, the Countess of Shaftesbury, but took a rather different approach. He took three stone jugs and filled them with the urine of the patient. He buried the jugs in the yard with a tile placed over their openings. Although done without the Countess's knowledge, Locke recorded that 'she had not from that time till now any of those violent nephritical pains she was wont to have'. This form of treatment operated on the basis of 'transference', where the disease was transferred to an animal or inanimate object and thereby removed from the body.

Mrs Stephen's Medicines

Some remedies developed great fame and prestige. In his diary for 1739, Richard Wilkes recorded that Alderman Fox of Coventry had been suffering from a suppression of the urine caused by kidney or bladder stones. Having tried numerous remedies Fox was convinced, against the wishes of his doctor, Dr Ingram, to take 'Mrs Steven's Medicines.' These, Wilkes claimed, raised his pulse and caused him to bleed at the nose and from haemorrhoids, and urinate much 'pale Water.' Numerous surgeons attempted to stop the excessive bleeding but it was to no avail and Fox died. Despite his evident distaste for the remedy, Wilkes recorded that Mrs Johanna Stevens was thought to have a medicine 'capable of dissolving the stone in [the] Bladder & Kidneys, many Persons as it was said having been cured by it, Parliament now purchased the Receipt off her for [£]5000'. This was evidently the case as a pamphlet produced in London in 1740 outlined 'A Most Excellent Cure for the Stone and Gravel as Published by Mrs. Joanna Stephens, for which Discovery she is allowed Five Thousand Pounds by Act of Parliament.' Likewise another pamphlet produced by 'Omnelio Pictarne, M.D.' claimed to unveil 'for the Public Good' the truth of Mrs Stephen's medicines. The acclaimed medicines turned out to be a powder made of eggshells and snails and some pills made of calcined snails, wild carrot seeds, burdock seeds, ash keys, rosehips and hawthorn berries, burnt to blackness and mixed with soap and honey.

Cutting for the Stone

For most patients suffering with kidney and bladder stones, a key focus of treatment was to avoid the surgeon's knife. If the stones were not passed when urinating or dissolved within the body, the only option left was to undergo surgical intervention. Lithotomy, contemporaneously known as 'cutting for the stone', was the operation both the French boy, described earlier, and Samuel Pepys endured. It was a grizzly and dangerous procedure that involved cutting either the penis or another part of the genital region to allow for the removal of stones with a variety of instruments like the crochet or forceps. The dangers of this operation ranged from damage to the urinary system to death. Many surgeons were adept at performing this operation, but it was still dangerous. Rivière lamented, 'how terrible it is, daily Experience will declare, because many die under that Operation'. Those who cut for the stone were known as lithotomists, and tales also circulated of wandering lithotomists and quacks who performed the surgery without adequate care. Robert Johnson noted in 1700 that the least some of these patients could expect was that the surgery wouldn't remove the root cause of the problem and they would be 'forced to endure that dreadful operation the second, and sometimes the third time, under which many have died, and others who recovered have never held their Urine.'

For the operation itself, the patient, if an adult, was shaved and sat upon a bed or a chair. Samuel Pepys recorded having his operation on his aunt's kitchen table in 1658 when he was a young man of 25. They were to draw their legs up and hold onto the heels, or as close as possible. If the surgery was performed on a child it was recommended that the surgeon's assistants were at hand to hold the child in place. The patient was tilted back slightly to give better access and an incision was made in the perineum to remove the stone. If a stone lodged in the urethra the incision might be made into the penis. The descriptions of these operations normally expected the patient to be male.

In the eighteenth century, barber-surgeon William Chesleden described a new method for cutting for the stone. St Thomas' Hospital employed Chesleden from 1720 as their specialist in this procedure. His method was set out in *A Treatise on the High Operation for the Stone* (1723) and was performed on a full bladder. This made for a much shorter and safer process and a much lower mortality rate.

As Johnson noted, surgery of this nature could cause lasting damage to the urinary tract. Jane Sharp warned that it could also damage the reproductive organs. She wrote in her 1671 *The Midwives Book*:

> to all that cut for the stone in the bladder, of what age soever they be who are cut; oftentimes in drawing forth the stone they so rend and tear the seed vessels, that such persons are never able to beget Children, they

may hatch the Cuckoo's Eggs, and keep other men's if they please, but they shall never get any themselves.

Sharp's hard words imply that men were routinely left infertile by this operation and so any children they thought they had fathered could not be their biological ones. It is tempting to speculate whether this happened to Pepys during his operation, since despite their hopes, he and his wife never had children. Pepys had many affairs and no children are thought to have come from these liaisons either. However, given the inherent dangers, it is little wonder that Pepys threw a house party on the anniversary of his operation each year to celebrate his survival and on-going good health.

As suggested here, the surgery could have lasting side effects and was not always straightforward. Given the complexity of the condition, there were some occasions that necessitated rather more *ad hoc* approaches. In *The Anatomy of Human Bodies* (1689), Isbrand van Diemerbroeck recorded the story of Lieutenant St George's 18-year-old son. The boy had been troubled from infancy with a gravel and was, at the time of seeing Diemerbroeck, 'so tormented with a Stone that stuck in both Ureters, that he knew not where to turn himself'. His treatment initially appeared successful and, having taken an apozem, his pain ceased and he voided a small stone as well as 'much Gravel.' However, Diemerbroeck noted that in the following month the patient was troubled again. This time the decoction he was taking moved the bladder stone in to the penis where it 'was so big it could not pass, but obstructed the Urine with most cruel Torture'. Diemerbroeck continued the story by relating that, faced with such incredible suffering in his son, 'which the Father not being able to bear, there being no surgeon to be sent for, with a Razor, made a small Wound underneath the Urinary Passage, where the Stone stuck; which done, the Stone spurted out, and the Urine followed in great quantity.'

Part Three

WHOLE BODY AILMENTS

Chapter 9

Agues: Frequent Fits of Fever

'I have an Ague on me, do you not see me shake?'

– Thomas Dekker

Samuel Jeake, a merchant from Rye, Sussex, meticulously recorded his own bouts of a condition known as ague in his diary. Jeake had radical Protestant leanings and believed that God ordained the events experienced in his daily life. But Jeake, slightly more unusually, also focused on astrology. He believed that God used the heavens and the influence of the stars to manipulate terrestrial events. In part, this accounts for his almost pedantic attentions to the minute details of his illnesses. It was crucial for Jeake's understandings of his health to know the moment at which his agues began, how long they lasted, their location in the body and their type. Thus in his diary we find successive and repetitive entries about agues and recurrent fevers, to which he attributed most of his experiences of ill health. For example, on 31 August 1670 he complained that 'I were taken with Quartan Ague [...] At first I was taken cold as usual; but when I were in bed, hot; accompanied with aches of the bones, & giddiness of the head. This Ague lasted 8 months'. On successive days after this he noted the symptoms he was experiencing. On 1 September he had a headache, painful bones, and 'oppression of the stomach' all day; on the third he suffered a second violent fit of the ague, on the sixth he had a third 'very bad' fit; on the ninth there was some reprieve as the fourth fit was 'so little that it could hardly be perceived'; by the twelfth things had deteriorated again and a fifth fit was 'accompanied with pain of the head & drowsiness'. Any change in his body from his normal expected sensations was therefore connected in his mind to the ague. By 2 May 1671 his diary reveals that he was now suffering from 'the 142nd and last fit; very mild & short'.

Put simply, an ague was a feverish fit or an intermittent fever, including malarial fevers. As Jeake's diary suggests, people defined agues by their type, length and recurrence. One that occurred daily was a quotidian ague, one that occurred every two days a quartan, every three days a tertian. Patients also experienced a range of symptoms alongside their fevers. In Jeake's case this included stomach problems and headaches, as well as sweating, shaking and on some occasions toothache. Writing at the beginning of the eighteenth century, Robert Johnston believed that several bodily changes could cause an ague. The first was sudden exposure to the cold, which closed the pores and prevented the flow of sweat out of the body; 'sweaty Vapours' held inside the body condensed and soured causing the outside of the body to experience chills and shivering. This blockage and disorder allowed the choler in the body to gain dominion and rarefy the blood, making the pulse stronger and quicker.

Alternatively, an internal phlegmy obstruction of the pancreas might be the cause of the disorder. Because the 'Juice of the *Pancreas*' was naturally inclined to be sour it would quickly grow acrimonious and acidic. Eventually this putrefying juice would break through the obstruction and rush into the duodenum, mixing with the choler found there. Johnston thought the resulting mixture stirred up a 'vicious effervescency, or preternatural Ferment' that triggered aguish symptoms: horror, shaking, chills, retching, and vomiting. The products of this damaging concoction circulated through the body, eventually reaching the heart and quickening the pulse; inducing further symptoms including heat, thirst, difficulty breathing, heartache, raving, and swooning. The thickness of the phlegm in the pancreas accounted for the various lulls between bouts, a thicker phlegm would hold back the pancreatic juices longer. Simon Mason, an apothecary writing on *The Nature of an Intermitting Fever and Ague* in 1745, astutely noted that these symptoms were not particular to this condition, perhaps explaining why 'aguish' was used to describe a range of symptoms and illnesses.

For early modern men and women the environment was a key factor in the prevalence and virulence of disease. Agues were no different. Medical writers advised that 'low, cold, marshy lands' and coastal towns in Kent, Essex and the Fens were harbingers of the disease because the air in these places contributed to the first cause of the disease. Simon Mason was clear that agues were common in Lincolnshire and the Isle of Ely because in these areas people often caught a cold. He was clear to point out though that 'they are to be met with in all Parts of our Kingdom', so living away from low-lying foggy, marshy areas was no guarantee of good health. These popular ideas about ill health and environment were born out by population figures. Historians have claimed that despite the colonisation and drainage of marshes in Kent, the population of these areas didn't rise. Disease was a factor in this. Long-term residents of these areas were somewhat protected from malarial and aguish problems. Yet newcomers were prone to these conditions and experienced higher mortality rates. Michael Zell has estimated that the conditions were so bad that between 1570 and 1670 the area lost about a third of its residents.

As Jeake's litany of fits suggests this was a commonly experienced ailment. While some of Jeake's fevers were mild and barely noticeable this was not the case for everyone. Yorkshire gentlewoman Alice Thornton wrote an auto-biography to justify herself to her detractors – she had been the subject of local gossip – and to put on record God's benevolence and kindness towards her. In the autobiography, Alice noted that numerous members of her family, herself included, experienced agues, some of which were severe. Just before their marriage, Alice's then fiancé suffered from an ague that caused him to be 'exceedingly ill'. Alice herself then fell into 'a most terrible shaking Ague lasting one quarter of a year, by fits each day twice in much violency, so that the sweats was great with faintings, being thereby [weakened] till I could not stand or go.' Alice recovered from this only to develop jaundice. Yet more tragically on 5 September 1656 Alice's daughter Elizabeth, who she affectionately called Betty, died from rickets and consumption. Alice noted, though, that these were 'gotten at first by an Ague'. Alice's brother John Ward also died from an ague and a fit of the stone.

In February 1661, Alice claimed that she was 'brought [...] very nigh to Death' with a cold and aguish temper. For five days she suffered vomiting, pain and weakness. Her doctor, Dr Wittie, gave her cordials and let blood, but on the night of 17 February she was convinced that it would be her last night on earth. Like many life writings from this era, Alice's focus was pre-dominantly on the ways in which her physical health allowed her to reaffirm her faith. In this case her aguish fever was particularly troubling because in her weakness and ill health she felt a despair and isolation from God and believed that she had been tempted by the devil. Overcoming this and being prepared to 'cast myself solely at his feet of mercy' and trust wholly in God for healing, Alice found both solace and health – she noted that in that very moment her symptoms began to abate.

Another early modern woman who suffered repeatedly from ague was the wife of dissenting minister Isaac Archer, and on 29 September 1667 Isaac noted in his diary that she had 'a quartane ague ever since August last, and her friends feared it might kill her, showing that it came from melancholy concerning my father's harshness, etc.' Isaac Archer's father didn't approve of his plans to marry Anne and father and son had fallen out badly. His father only learned that he had been blamed for Anne's melancholy-induced ague a few months later and was furious; on 25 November Isaac recorded that he 'wrote me a chiding letter'. The next spring saw Isaac too come down with ague, tertian this time. He was staying with his in-laws where 'they took great care of me'. Isaac was puzzled as to why he'd become ill, and wrote:

> *I know not how it came about; for I have designed it not; in my first fit*
> *I spoke much to my wife concerning religion, heaven, the way thither,*
> *and many passages concerning myself, and my former life, what comfort*
> *I now found, and what joy I should have in case God should take me*
> *away.*

Being ill had given Isaac the chance for a heart-to-heart with his wife, which he decided was the lesson God was giving in making him ill. He had mentioned in his diary before about his 'youthful desires' and how they had been cured by marriage, and that he carried a lot of guilt up until this point for them. He had five fits of ague but pronounced himself cured on 2 May, imputing the experience as an occasion for spiritual cleansing, and like Alice Thornton, for coming closer to God.

Others experienced severe agues that left them weak for some time afterwards. While travelling across France, John Locke, the physician and philosopher, was struck down with a severe fit of ague that delayed his progress for six weeks and left him feeling under the weather for several months. The severity of symptoms is, of course, in some ways subjective and eminent physician Thomas Sydenham dismissed Locke's as 'no other than what are usual after agues'. Given that he felt easily tired, Locke was possibly less than impressed with Sydenham's advice that exercise, particularly horse riding, would be beneficial to his recovery.

Cures and Recovery

When he fell sick with the 'grudging of an Ague' and then a tertian fever in August 1653, John Evelyn utilised phlebotomy and purges to redress the imbalance of humours in his body. His treatments took thirteen days whereupon, he recorded, 'it pleased God to restore me'. Like John Locke, Evelyn felt that this bout of illness had 'in this short time extremely weakened' him, even to the point that he could not attend church. Modern readers might infer that treatments like bloodletting can have only added to this fatigue.

Simon Mason claimed that provoking diarrhoea often helped ease a fever because it removed morbific (diseased) matter from the body. He noted that many patients experienced respite from the symptoms of a fever upon evacuation. This could help ward off an impending fit and change the length of time between fits because 'removing the Matter from the Blood is taking away the Cause, and according to the Quantity of Matter taken from the Blood' a different length of intermission of symptoms might be gained. Not everyone agreed with Mason's favoured method of treatment. When James Hervey was treated for an ague in the early eighteenth century his mother complained 'I don't find that either the bleeding, blistering, or purging gives him any relief'. Another popular method of treatment was to remove this offending matter by provoking sweating. Mason complained that several of his patients pushed for this method of bodily evacuation over bleeding. The handwritten recipe book of Lady Ayscough recommended 'a handful of Marigolds flowers and all an handful of holy thistle' beaten and strained to remove the 'purest of the juice' made into a posset of ale with sugar. This, she wrote, will 'cast him [the patient] into a sweat'.

Mason also wrote in his treatise that some people used charms and amulets to cure agues. The recipe book of Edward and Katherine Kidder included one remedy that might be considered a charm. Under an entry entitled 'A cure for the ague', the author wrote:

when the Judas led Christ to the place of execution they said he had a fever but he answered he had neither ague, nor fever and whoever did were these words written about their right arm should never have ague nor fever

Those living in England's marshlands had their own ritualistic remedies. One was for the patient to cut several rods, according to the hour when the fit occurred – so a fit beginning at 9 am required nine rods. The rods were burned individually while the patient or medical practitioner repeated, 'as the rods burn, let the ague burn too'. As we have seen in other chapters, belief in treatments like this one was based upon the idea of transference and symbolism – transferring the disease to the rods, as they were burned so the disease would be destroyed. Another treatment that worked in this way was to tie a lock of hair to a tree and then wrench yourself free, leaving the lock and the ague on the tree.

The Jesuits' Powder

Jesuit missionaries were an important conduit for the transmission of medical and scientific knowledge gathered in the Americas. One new drug that found its way back to Europe in the 1630s was cinchona bark, which contains quinine. It was known as 'Peruvian bark', 'Jesuits' Bark' or 'Jesuits' Powder' in recognition of the fact the Society of Jesus were the first to bring it to the attention of European medics. It also reflected the fact that the Society dominated its supply and distribution.

The drug was tested in Rome in 1645 on feverish hospital patients, and the Society distributed the drug free of charge to the poor. The trials, according to some historians, were part of a well-orchestrated campaign by the Society to promote the sale of the drug. Some medics were convinced by the efficacy of the bark, both in fighting agues and in treating other diseases. Thomas Sydenham, known as the modern Hippocrates, generally advocated a policy of non-intervention in curing disease. He believed that nature would work to remedy the condition herself without interference from physicians. Yet even he promoted a select number of remedies – including the bark. He believed that it was a 'specific' suited particularly to the treatment of agues. After his fit in France, Sydenham wrote a letter to John Locke outlining the appropriate use of the Peruvian bark as a cure.

Dr Willis's Practice of Physick from 1684 claimed that two drams of bark beaten to a powder and infused in sack, a sweet Spanish wine, for two hours should be given to the patient while in bed. The potion made in this way would prevent a fit, if it was taken before the first fit started. It would then also work to prevent subsequent fits so that it would seem as if the disease was cured. However, it was a temporary measure as after 'twenty or thirty days' the fits would start again and a new dose would be needed. Thomas Willis died in 1675, but this posthumous collection of his works did not include the suggestion that another author had tampered with the information, suggesting to buyers that they were a faithful rendition of Willis's medical works. If this is true, Willis could not explain how the effects of this drug came about. He recounted: 'If it be demanded, concerning the Nature of this Bark, and the virtue in suppressing the fits of Intermitting Fevers, it is not to be dissembled, that 'tis very difficult to explicate the causes of these kinds of effects, and the manner of working [...] a general Reason is not to be rightly fitted'.

Not everyone was in favour of the novel wonder drug from the new world, and at various moments Sydenham too shared the concerns that others had about the Peruvian bark. A particular concern for English Protestants was that the drug was associated with 'Popery' and Catholicism. Some feared that the drug was a Catholic plot, a poison, designed to rid the world of Protestants. Oliver Cromwell refused to use the treatment when he fell ill of an ague in 1658 because of its association with the Jesuits. Another concern was that the drug's cost motivated some disreputable sellers to produce fake and adulterated versions of the medicine. Sir Hans Sloane discovered, for example, that some people were preparing the bark of the cherry tree for sale as cinchona by soaking it in a tincture of aloes. This gave it the requisite bitter taste to appear to be cinchona, but was likely to cause diarrhoea in those who consumed it.

Robert Talbor, who had trained as an apothecary in Cambridge was one of those who helped to popularise the drug. In the preface to his medical text *Pyretologia, a Rational Account of the Cause & Cure of Agues* (1672), he explained how he had developed his skill and knowledge in curing the disease:

> *I planted myself in Essex near to the seaside, in a place where Agues are the epidemical diseases, where you will find but few persons but either are, or have been afflicted with a tedious Quartan: In this place I lived some years, making the best use of my time I could, for the improving my knowledge; curiously observing all symptoms, Diagnostics and Prognostics; by which observations, and the assistance of my reason (God blessing my endeavours) I have attained to a perfect knowledge of the cure of the most inveterate and pertinacious Agues.*

After all his experimentation Talbor developed a successful fever medicine, which he kept a secret throughout his career. Charles II appointed him as a physician-in-ordinary after a French nobleman explained to him Talbor's success and in July 1678 Talbor was knighted. Talbor then travelled to Europe where he healed the dauphin of France who was suffering a pernicious fever. Charles II himself caught a fever and eventually, despite scepticism and opposition from other physicians, was successfully given cinchona. Talbor's success with the drug helped cement its position as a specific remedy for fever and swept away concerns about its origins. After Talbor's death the French King had details of his remedy published, revealing that it was indeed cinchona, mixed with spices and wine.

Chapter 10

Cancer: In the Crab's Claws

'the Wolf and Canker (which / On her make fat their dreadful Luxury)'
– Joseph Beaumont

The absolute importance of keeping the humours in good balance was never more starkly exemplified than when it came to cancers. An over-abundance of black bile, also known as Devil's balm because of the black thoughts it induced, was held to be the prime cause of cancer. In 1565, *A Most Excellent and Learned Work of Chirurgerie* translated by a John Hall from the thirteenth-century writings of Lanfranc of Milan (1250-1306), explained that there were two types of cancer: ulcerated or non-ulcerated. Non-ulcerous cancer was 'made by growing even from the beginning of putrefied melancholy [...] At which time it beginneth to show like a Lupin, and sometime it groweth like a great Melon.' Otherwise, 'it is made by conversion of a hard apostume [abscess], coming of natural melancholy not corrupted.' Ulcerated cancers, known as cankers, were thought to come from badly healed wounds, whereas non-ulcerated ones were trickier to diagnose early. Cankers were detectable because they stank badly and if the sore was washed with a lye soap, then fluid like 'slimy spittle' ran out. However, these ulcerated sores were a non-healing wound and not what would nowadays be associated with cancer.

The Hippocratic corpus had named the disease, or set of diseases, after the Greek for crab. As Philemon Holland, who translated Roman historian Pliny's *Natural Histories* into English in 1601, described, a true '*Cancer* is a swelling or sore coming of melancholy blood, about which the veins appear of a black or swart colour, spread in manner of a Crayfish claws'. In the later seventeenth century William Salmon's *Synopsis Medicinæ* described how 'Cancer is a hard round Tumour blue or blackish having pain and beating'. Describing cancer as a crab served to make the disease seem, unlike humoural descriptions tended to, like an external force attacking the body. In particular medical writers noted that cancer caught the flesh and wouldn't release it, like being caught in a crab's pincers. Philip Barrough argued, for example, that cancer was 'very hardly pulled away from those members, which it doth lay hold on, as the sea crab doth, who obstinately doth cleave to that place which it once hath apprehended.' Medical writers throughout the era also referred to cancer as a worm that burrowed and forced its way into the flesh and caused decay and corruption. Cancer gnawed and ate at the flesh. Likewise, medical writers described the disease in predatory terms, calling it a wolf, as it was cruel, fierce and ravenous in its destruction of the body. Adam Thomas's 1615 religious treatise used the image of cancer as a metaphor for corruption in the church and mentioned that it was 'vulgarly the *wolfe*', suggesting that colloquially this was what people called cancers. Cancers in the legs were most often called this, and indeed, the short-lived newspaper *British Apollo* ('Curious Amusements for the Ingenious') noted in an edition from 1709 that 'What is call'd by [...] Surgeons a Wolf, is a sort of Cancerous Ulcer, more properly so called when in the Legs'.

A Feminine Disease?

Whereas, as we have seen, women were less likely to develop diseases like the stone because of their wetter humoral makeup, women were considered to be more at risk of cancer. This was particularly true if their periods stopped, since one of the jobs of menstruation was to draw with it other toxic matter from the body. Stopped menstruation was considered to be the primary cause of breast cancer, for example. In that case, excess and toxic matter travelled via the 'epigastric' venous connection, which was thought to link the womb to the breast. In her 1671 midwifery guide, Jane Sharp explained that 'when the Menstrual blood runs back to the breasts, this will soon become a Cancer'. It wasn't just suppressed menstruation that left women vulnerable to breast cancer, however, as Oxford physician Thomas Willis explained, 'when a small hurt happens to the Breast of a Woman, a *Cancer* follows'. Knocking the breast caused melancholic humours to pool there causing cancerous growth.

Early diagnosis was difficult, as Sharp noted: 'A Cancer that comes naturally undiscerned, is hardly known at first, being no greater than a pea, and daily increaseth with roots spreading, and Veins about it' by the time it is visible to the human eye 'when the skin is eaten through it becomes a loathsome Ulcer: the Matter is black, and the lips are hard; it is scarce curable, because it is bred of black burnt blood that is malign' and the cancer was sure to spread.

'As Good as a Rotten Apple': Non-surgical Cures for Cancer

A sixteenth-century book of cures, *The Treasury of Health* (1553), which claimed to be a translation of a book of that name by Pope XXI (d. 1277), suggested that:

Olive leaves stamped with honey heals the Cancer in the yard [penis]
or elsewhere, also let the place be washed with warm vinegar and dried
with a linen cloth, sprinkle thereon powder of galls, do this thrice a day
and it shall heal it perfectly in short space.

Similarly, a posthumous version of William Bullein's *Herbal*, called *Bulleins*
Bulwarke of Defence Against all Sickness, Soreness and Wounds (1579), argued
that 'Nothing prevaileth more against the Cancer, than the juice of Ivy, tem-
pered with clarified Honey, & Wine sodden together'.

Treating cancer was hard, and *A Most Excellent and Learned Work of*
Chirurgerie explained that it was best to try and purge it from the body since
partial removals were pointless:

The first general rule in the cure of a Cancer, is, that it is never perfectly
healed, unless it be utterly extirpated, with all his roots. And therefore of
this rule springeth a second necessary rule, that it ought not to be cured
by cauteries [...] *except it be in such a place where it may utterly be had*
away. If therefore the Cancer not ulcerate, be in a place replete with
veins, sinews, muscles and arteries, as in the neck, or in the mammil-
liaries [sic], *or such like: see then that thou enterprise not to ripe it,*
nor break it, nor cut it, nor cauterize it: but purge the body with some
medicine, that purgeth choler.

At the same time as purging the body of its excess black choler, patients
needed to manage their diet and eat a temperate menu, abstaining from
meat, cheese, pepper, and all the foodstuffs thought likely to heat the body.
The lump should be dressed with a salve designed to stop it becoming ulcerated. If it did become ulcerated then this book saw palliative care as the only
option: 'But it may be palliated by anointing it with the unguent of *Tatiae*
and the diet aforesaid: and so may the patient's life be prolonged.' It is likely
that this palliative idea was behind the eminent surgeon Alexander Read's
decision to treat Mrs Culpeper with an ointment of red lead known for its
cooling and drying properties. Discussing his mother's illness in *The London*
Dispensatory (1653), Nicholas Culpeper claimed the cure was entirely ineffective. He wrote that, despite the fact that the treatment was applied before
the cancer broke, it had done as much good 'as though he had applied a
rotten Apple' to it. It has to be said though, that eminent scientist Robert
Boyle's recommendation in 1693 to treat breast cancer was that one should
'*Take of the Warts that grow on the hinder Legs of a (Stone) Horse, dry them*

gently, till you can reduce them to a Powder, of which you may give half a Dram for a Dose in any convenient Vehicle' doesn't sound any more effective.

Surgical Interventions

The severity of cancer and the terrible effects it wrought on the body encouraged practitioners of all kinds to seek a cure. These were not simply the dressings and ointments previously discussed, but drastic surgical interventions. As the 1565 text *A Most Excellent and Learned Work of Chirurgerie* explained, partial removal or cauterisation would not cure a cancer, only a total removal could hope to do this. Attempts to do this became increasingly prominent in the treatment of breast cancer. As might be expected in an era before anaesthetics and antiseptics, mastectomy, like all operations, was both excruciating and dangerous. An English edition of Charles Gabriel Le Clerc's French text *The Complete Surgeon* explained the procedure:

> *The sick Patient being laid in Bed, the Surgeon takes the Arm on the side of the Cancer, and lifts it upward and backward, to give more room to the Tumour; then having passed a Needle with a very strong Thread through the bottom of the Breast, he cuts the Thread to take away the Needle, and passeth the Needle again into the Breast, to cause the Threads to cross one another. Afterward these four ends of the Threads are tied together, to make a kind of Handle to take off the Tumour, which is cut quite round to the Ribs with a very sharp Razor.*

Once removed, the wound was dressed with astringent powders, plasters and bandages. Going under the knife was still no guarantee of a cure. Mr Monro, an anatomist in Edinburgh, supposedly claimed that of sixty cancers he had seen removed, only four patients remained free from the disease after two years. He also noted that the disease did not always return to the same part of the body, and was often 'more violent' and progressed much more quickly than in those patients who had not been operated on.

An alternative method was to try and remove the cancerous tissue using caustics that would corrode the offending flesh. By the late eighteenth century, one surgeon at least was cautioning against it as 'too cruel for any surgeon to practice'. William Rowley was the surgeon at St John's Hospital in Holborn and he lamented that it was the preserve of quacks to call all diseases of the breasts cancers, and by using their caustics cause patients much 'misery'. Patients' willingness to undergo such treatments reflected the poor prognosis for the disease, but Rowley claimed that in such cases where 'cure cannot be accomplished by any means', a compassionate and sensible practitioner would employ palliative treatments to achieve 'considerable improvements', such as those discussed above.

Cashing In? Advertising a Cure

Sometimes healers advertised their cures in the back of other books or pamphlets. One Dr Vanderplase took out an advert in the back of the records of the proceedings of the Old Bailey for 6 December 1710. This took the form of a testimonial from John Bragnell who was quoted as saying:

> I John Bragnell, living in King street, in the Parish of Wapping, Stepney, being affected with a Cancer in my Face, which did eat away my Nose, and a great Part of my Face, so that my Life was despaired of; but hearing of the great Cures daily performed in this, and other deplorable Diseases, by Dr. Vanderplase, in Upper Shadwell, over against New Gravel Lane, I addressed myself to him; who has, with the Help of God, made me a Perfect and Sound Man. I desire this Certificate may be published for the Good of others. John Bragnell.

In case this inspired the reader to follow suit, the doctor's particulars were given immediately below, 'The Dr. may be advised with every Day at Yates's Coffee House, in the Paved Alley in Leadenhall Market, at Two or three of the Clock.'

In a similar way, a Dr Jones of Hatton Garden released a small seven-page book of 'his cures', those he had claimed to cure, specifically dated to 18 April 1673, along with details of when he was available for consultations. His patients included:

> Elizabeth Theson of Newington Butts in Blackman street in Southwark, in Lamb Alley, of a Cancer in her Breast almost as big as a man's head, and I consumed it away without cutting, or putting her to any pain, or hindering her business.

This type of unspecified cure, probably the cure-all pill he aimed to sell at the end of the booklet, went against all the teachings about how to approach a cancer. But, not content at one breast cancer anecdote, Jones told a lengthier story:

the wife of William Thomas in Cock Lane, going out of Care Street to Nicholas Street in Bristol, [who I cured] of a Cancer in her left breast and side, when they that had her in hand gave her off for a dead woman [that is to say, those who were caring for her declared she was ill beyond hope of a cure], *the Distemper being so bad with hardness of red, yellow, and black colours, which was very sad to behold, and they every day put in a Tent between her Ribs quite into her body, about the length and bigness of a man's finger, so that I judge the end of the Tent must needs go within an inch of her heart; she had also a continual Fever attending on her, so that there could not anything be expected but death, I presently caused the Tent to be laid by, and I never applied Tent nor Instrument, but gave her present ease, and cured her in about nine or ten weeks time, with God's help.*

A tent is a roll of fabric used to keep a wound open and so let it drain and heal, and was the standard treatment for a sore like this. The cures Mrs Thomas's previous doctors were attempting were extremely invasive, making Jones' miracle pill all the more appealing in contrast.

In reality, and away from the hyperbole of the quack doctors, prognosis wasn't good in a true cancer. As Jane Sharp commented, womb cancer was seldom seen but if found was incurable. Cancer seems to have been less common in the past than now and this is due to an ageing population. The longer someone lives, the more likely it is that they will develop cancer. In the Bill of Mortality for the August week at the height of the Great Plague in 1665, just two people were thought to have died of cancer, the same as had died from drowning, and this is a tiny number compared with the 353 who died of fever, or even the seventy-four from 'griping guts', for example. The main difference between the experience of cancer then and now is that cancers were much more visible: they were not fully diagnosable, even when suspected, until the tumour and its brackish blood supply had broken the skin.

Chapter 11

Diabetes: The Pissing Evil

'Nor yet of Salt, and Sugar, sweet and smart, / Both when we list,
to water we convert'
– Anne Bradstreet

iabetes in the early modern era was a startling, dangerous illness. This is revealed in the descriptions used by medical writers to introduce people to the disease. In 1694 John Peachi, a French doctor and extra licentiate of the Royal College of Physicians from 1683, published a short pamphlet advocating a new herb 'perigua' as a remedy for the disease. He was trying to sell his new magnificent remedy and so was inclined to exaggeration, but he opened with the following description:

> *that sad and deplorable Distemper known by the Name of* Diabetes, *or making abundance of Water, which quickly Ends in Death, and con-temns the best of our* European *Remedies.*

A later eighteenth-century author concurred but was even more succinct in his declaration that the disease 'generally proves mortal, in spite of the Force of Medicine.' A key feature of diabetes was its resistance to medical intervention.

As well as being startling, it was also a disease on the rise. Medical writers in the eighteenth century argued that Galen had scarcely treated two patients for the condition, but now it was much more common. Several famous people are thought to have suffered from the condition including Cardinal Wolsey, Henry VIII's first chief minister, and the Elizabethan Lord Chancellor Sir Christopher Hatton, of whom one chronicler lamented that his disease was as 'unmannerly as [it was] troublesome'. Narcissus Luttrell noted in his diary in 1690 that 'the earl of Gainsborough died lately of a diabetes'. Baptist Noel Wriothesley, the second earl of Gainsborough was only 29 when he died so, if Luttrell's observation is correct, it seems diabetes claimed him at a very young age. Yet despite dramatic descriptions and famous victims, a Bill of Mortality published in London detailing baptisms and burials between December 1687 and December 1688 claimed that only four people had died of diabetes. This suggests that disease had a rather limited impact, given that over 1,300 died in the same period from smallpox and measles, and nearly 1,500 died from 'Teeth'.

The Pissing Evil

Although the name is the same, coming into English directly from Latin where it means 'siphon' because of the excessive water flow it occasions, and the symptoms being very similar, men and women in this era experienced diabetes rather differently. Predominantly, it was understood as a disease of the urine and the kidneys, and some medical texts called it the 'pissing evil' – although it was different from cystitis or 'strangury' as it was known, which was painful and slow urination. Medical writers happily summarised the disease as, for example, John Johnston did: '*A Diabetes is a most quick and plentiful pissing of the drink unchanged, arising from the intense attractive faculty of the kidneys, and afflicting with a strong perpetual thirst*', but some broke the disorder down into different types. Michael Ettmüller claimed that there were two versions of the disease: genuine and spurious. Genuine diabetes was where a patient urinated liquids that had not undergone any 'alteration' in the body, whereas spurious diabetes was where the quantity of urine vastly exceeded the amount of liquids consumed by the patient.

Medical practitioners and writers did not agree about what caused the condition. Johnston thought that an 'afflux of sharp and biting humours' could trigger overactive kidney function. However, he also noted that large veins and large ureters could cause diabetes, as well as heat in the liver, pestilential fevers and a weakness of the stomach's retentive faculty. Ettmüller split these causes between his two types of illness – with genuine diabetes being the result of large, lax vessels, and spurious diabetes being caused by sharp, violent ferments. Charles Perry, writing in 1741, more firmly believed that the problem resided in a defective digestive system. This allowed the liquid parts of food and drink to move into the blood stream too quickly, however, as it had not been properly digested, it moved equally as rapidly into the kidneys and then out of the body. The frequent release of fluids from the body that typified this condition was used as a metaphor to describe other forms of 'incontinence' notably gossiping and revealing other people's secrets. As one aphorism stated: 'Revealing secrets is, by *Sir Richard Steele*, called a diabetic passion, a kind of incontinence of the mind, that retains nothing; perpetually, and almost insensibly, evacuating all.'

A Drunkard's Disease

Several writers explained that excessive drinking of diuretics was a contributing factor to this condition. John Peachi claimed that he 'knew a Clergyman who drank abundance of Tea, and whatever Friends came to visit, he must drink three or four dishes with them', which 'at length it brought him into this Distemper'. John Ovington's book describing the origins and virtues of tea, dedicated to the Countess of Grantham in 1699, contradicted this claim however, pointing out that if tea really was a 'parent' to the disease, then 'all the *Eastern Nations,* especially *China, India,* and Jamaica, must needs be sorely afflicted' because tea was commonly consumed in those nations. That this was not the case proved, Ovington argued, that tea was not a cause of the disease.

Instead of blaming tea, in 1695 John Pechey claimed that the early modern predilection for imbibing alcohol was one of the reasons why the disease was becoming ever more common. He wrote: 'This Disease was so rare amongst the Ancients, that many famous Physicians made no mention of it; but in our Age, where excessive Drinking has been, especially of Wine, so much used, there are many Instances of it.' The association of diabetes with heavy drinking allowed for moral reproach of those who fell ill, and perhaps gave medical writers ammunition in condemning the lack of restraint they saw in people's attitudes to alcohol.

A posthumous translation of Oxford physician Thomas Willis's works noted that an acquaintance of his developed the disease by drinking too much 'Rhenish Wine' (wine produced in the region of the Rhine River). An eighteenth-century medical writer retold the story embellishing that the patient used 'Rhenish Wine for his ordinary drink twenty days together, [and thereby] contracted an incurable *Diabetes,* of which he died within a month.' As this story suggests, the association with alcoholic intake lasted throughout the seventeenth and into the eighteenth century, although some started to question the types of drinking at fault. A short pamphlet, *A Mechanical Enquiry into the Nature, Causes, Seat, and Cure of the Diabetes,* produced in 1745, argued that while drinking strong alcoholic beverages to excess could cause diabetes, habitual drinking of alcohol did not cause the condition.

The Taste Test

The disorder, medical texts suggest, was relatively easy to diagnose through a patient's thirst and constant desire to urinate. Overwhelmingly it was the quantity of urine that revealed the nature of a patient's disease. In some cases these quantities could stretch the imagination. One text published in 1683 and attributed to Edward Madeira Arrais claimed that a 12-year-old maid, 'lying sick of a *Diabetes*', turned not only her food and water into urine, but the 'Ambient Air' drawn in through respiration. Thus she managed to urinate 'thirty six pounds of Water every day', even though she only ate 7lbs of meat and drink, and only weighed 150lbs herself. The author concluded that because her condition lasted 'threescore days', she must have shed 740lbs of urine, 'much more than the Weight of the Maid [herself], if she had even been all dissolved into Urine'.

However, as had been noted since ancient times, the sweet taste of their urine also easily identified 'Diabetical' patients. As Michael Ettmüller put it, 'the Symptoms of the spurious *Diabetes* are the crudity, thinness, and sweet taste of the Urine, with a fat Scum swimming upon it'. The sweetness was of a specific kind, Daniel Turner explained in *Ancient Physician's Legacy* (1733), it was 'like Water wherein Honey had been dissolved.' Uroscopy, or the examination of urine, was still a widely used diagnostic tool. Physicians not only looked at sediments in the urine and its colour to diagnose diseases but would taste the liquid, usually by dipping a finger into the liquid then licking it, to assess its composition. In addition to being sweet, some medical authors also suggested that the urine of diabetics was thin, pale and had an agreeable smell.

Curing Diabetes

The disease, like many others in this era, was thought to be easier to cure in certain bodies than others. John Peachi claimed that the 'Disease is very dangerous in Old men' because their natural heat was already decayed, but was also 'hard to Cure in young Men' because they 'will seldom be obliged to observe Rules' of treatment. Their lack of self-control meant their disease was likely to continue and worsen despite their treatment.

Medical writers generally lamented that the disease was difficult to cure and often led to death. Michael Ettmüller's book noted that, if the symptoms of diabetes 'follow immoderate Labour, Venery, or Chronic Fevers, 'tis uncurable'. As William Buchan put it, in diabetes: 'The strength fails, the appetite decays, and the flesh wastes away till the patient is reduced to skin and bone.' But one or two medical writers included observations of patients who had survived the disease. John Pechey wrote about one nobleman who 'fell into a desperate Diabetes' and 'voided a Gallon and an half of clear Urine, that was almost as sweet as Honey, in the space of a Night and a Day'. Despite a great thirst, a fever, and weakness of his whole body, the patient recovered. This was not permanent though, as Pechey explained that the man 'fell into the same Disease again' after being 'well a long time'. It was clearly a disease that, as suggested, tested the abilities of medical practitioners.

Despite the pessimistic outlook, numerous remedies and medicines were suggested in a range of texts. Those who believed the disorder was caused by poor digestion recommended heating and 'corroborating', strengthening, the stomach to promote good digestion. More broadly William Buchan recommended a diet that included rice, milk, and shellfish, particularly oysters and crabs. Likewise, physicians recommended that patients consume foods that would counteract the acidity in the blood that contributed to the disease, and watery and cooling foods that would replenish the moisture being lost through urination.

Numerous printed treatises suggested remedies that might ease the condition. Nicholas Culpeper's translation of the *Pharmacopoeia Londinensis* (1653), a list of the best-known cures, recommended the rather unappetising burnt bladder of a sheep or goat. *Medicinal Experiments* (1693) similarly recommended baked sheep's bladder pulverised into a powder. It is likely that these remedies functioned through the idea of sympathy, or the doctrine of signatures, where the likeness of a plant or animal product to the affected part of the body made it a relevant remedy – in this case consuming a bladder for a disease of the bladder and urine. Charles Perry, best known for his travel writing but also a medic, recommended a decoction made of lime taken with cinnamon and the roots of tormentil (a herbaceous perennial plant of the rose family) in his 1741 book of diseases, which was perhaps slightly more palatable.

Several families collected recipes to make diabetes remedies in the home as well. They recorded these under several variant spellings of the disease including 'dyabetis', and 'Diabetus'. The seventeenth-century book of Elizabeth Godfrey, for example, recommended a mixture of the powder of burnt hartshorn, roots of great comfrey, and dried and sliced water lilies, boiled with a crust of bread. Once mixed and boiled, the concoction was sweetened with six ounces of 'pearled sugar'. The patient drank a quarter of a pint of the resultant mixture every night, two hours after supper. A far less complex remedy was suggested in the book of Joanna Saint John who recommended 'A Hot two penny Loaf eat it all up at one time.'

In the eighteenth century the Bristol Waters became a particularly popular remedy. Charles Perry noted that they were 'accounted a Specific in this

Distemper'. *The Lady's Companion* (1743) wrote that 'The *Bristol* Water is such a known Specific in this Complaint, that the Use of that is almost all that need be prescribed in that Case' (although it then went on to recommend quince marmalade and Peruvian bark as well). None of these cures were likely to be very effective in a disease caused by insulin deficiency, and it seems likely that diabetes was on the rise in the period.

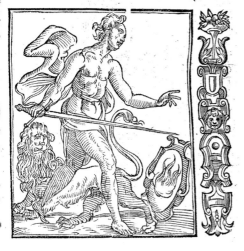

Yellow choler, also known as bile (hence bilious): 'The hot and dry humour. People with this as their dominant humour were often thought to have a fiery temperament. It is linked to summer and to fire.' (Wellcome Library, London)

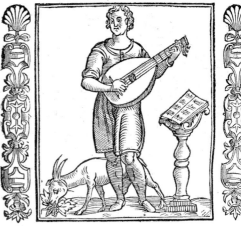

Blood: 'Hot and moist humour associated with childhood, Spring and the element air.' (Wellcome Library, London)

FLEMMATICO PER L'ACQVA.

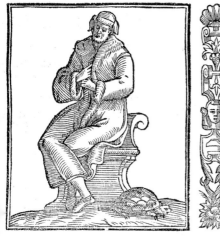

gm: 'Cold and moist, often ciated with old age. It is linked to lement water and to the winter n.' (Wellcome Library, London)

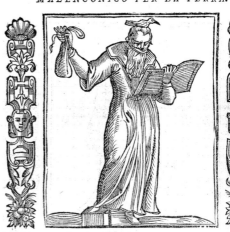

Melancholy or Black Bile:
'Cold and Dry. Linked with
Autumn and the earth.'
(Wellcome Library, London)

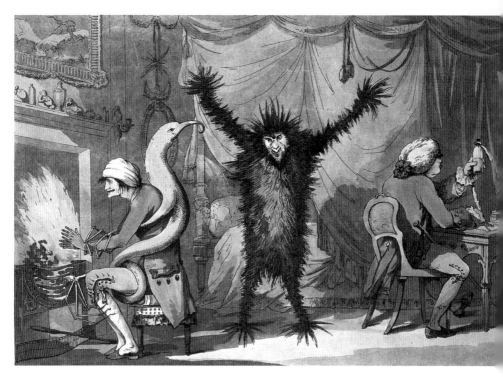

Ague: 'Fever, represented as a frenzied beast, stands racked in the centre of a room, while a blue monster, representing ague, ensnares his victim by the fireside; a doctor writes prescriptions to the right, 1788.' (Wellcome Library, London)

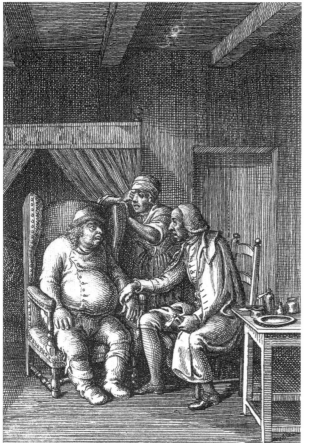

Dropsy: 'Johann Gottfried Mathes, a "natural healer", taking the pulse of a patient suffering from the dropsy, 1784. (Wellcome Library, London)

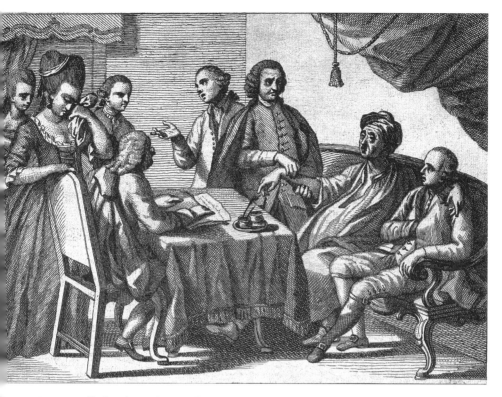

Dropsy: 'A man suffering from dropsy dictating his will whilst a physician takes his pulse, he is surrounded by his wife and friend.' (Wellcome Library, London)

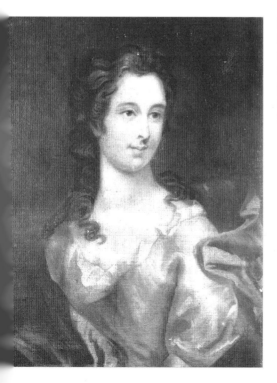

Smallpox: 'Portrait of Lady Mary Wortley Montague whose early support for inoculation for smallpox pioneered the preventative method in the eighteenth century.' (Wellcome Library, London)

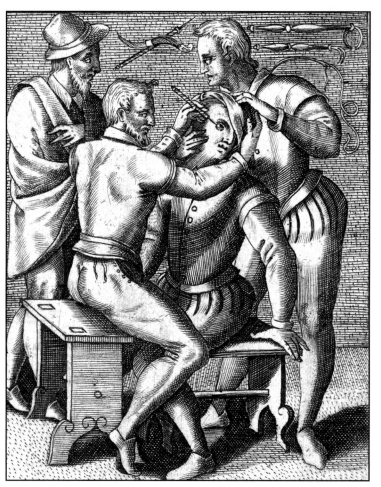

Eyes: 'The patient is held in place while a operation is perform on his eye, 1594.' (Wellcome Library, London)

'Seventeenth-centu eye-glasses with he rims and hinged me bridge in cardboard case with initials "I.B."' (Wellcome Library, London)

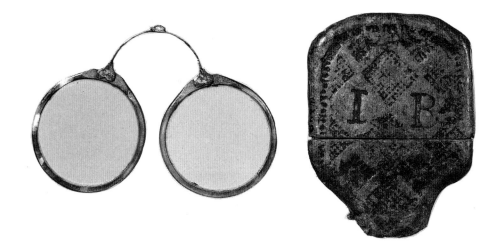

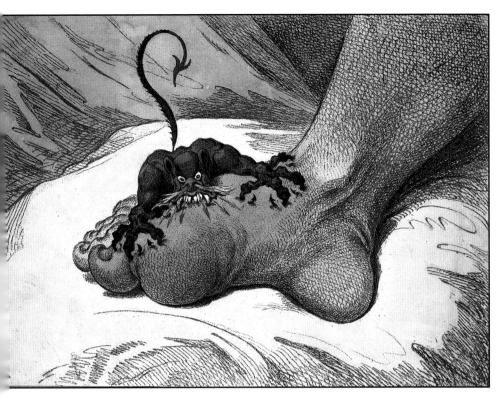

nes Gillray, "The Gout", 1799.' (Wellcome Library, London)

o gout sufferers, the richer carried on a litter, the poorer using crutches; (background) a man
g treated for gout, 1559.' (Wellcome Library, London)

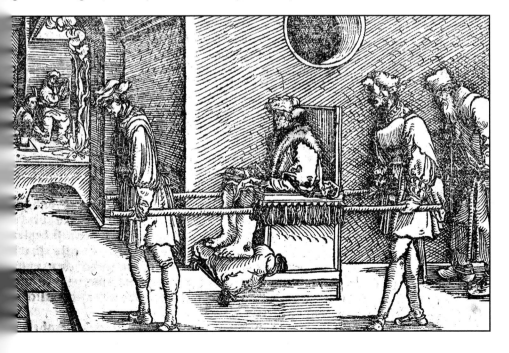

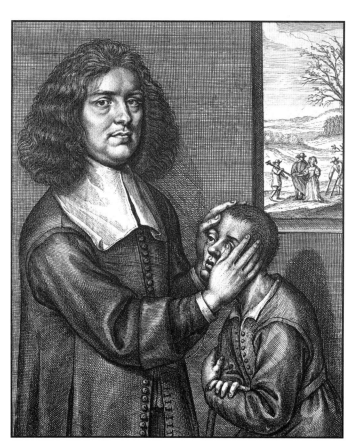

'Portrait of Valentine
Greatrakes laying on h
hands. The window in
the corner shows severa
successful "cures", c.16
(Wellcome Library, Lo▮

Headaches: 'One patien
lies still as trepanning i▮
performed on his skull.
Another apprehensive
looking man sits beside
being prepared to under
the same operation, 159
(Wellcome Library, Lo▮

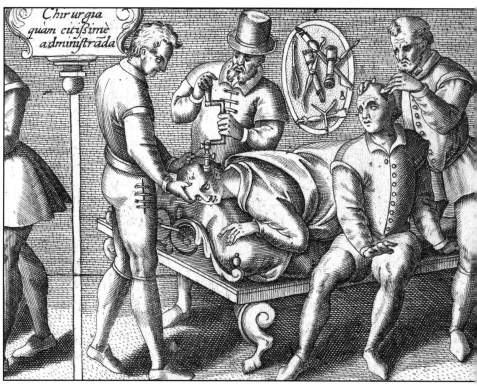

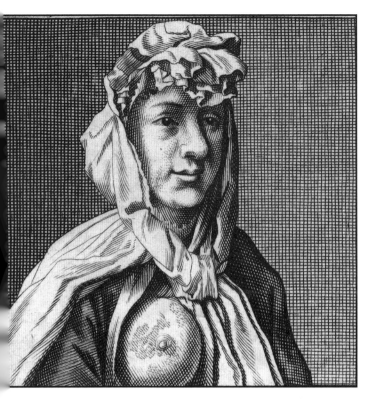

Cancer: 'Elizabeth Hopkins of Oxford, showing a breast with cancer which was removed by Sir William Read, 1700.' (Wellcome Library, London)

Infestations: 'A drawing of a flea from Robert Hooke's Micrographia, 1665.' (Wellcome Library, London)

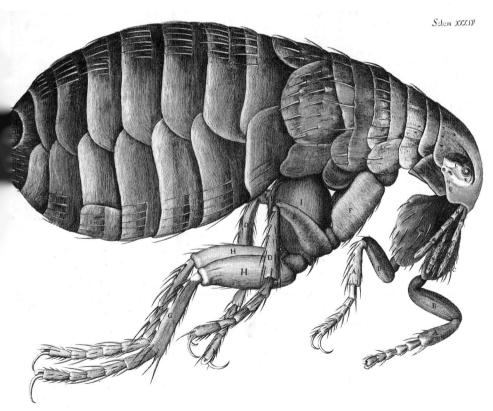

Schem XXXIV

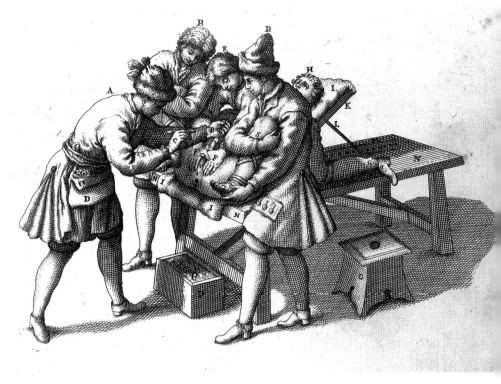

Kidney and Bladder Stones: 'Lithotomy (surgical removal of a stone or stones from the urinary tract) being performed, 1707.' (Wellcome Library, London)

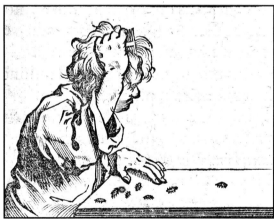

'Boy combing lice out of hair, 1639.' (Wellcome Library, London)

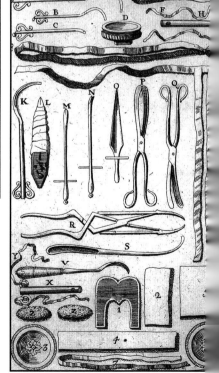

'Instruments used in a lithotomy, 1708.' (Wellcome Library, London)

'Charles II touching a patient for the king's evil (scrofula) surrounded by courtiers, clergy and general public.' (Wellcome Library, London)

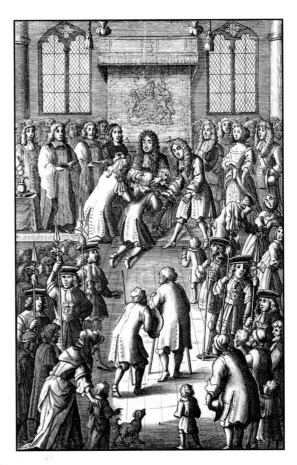

Plague: 'Bill of Mortality from August 15–22, 1665, at the height of the Great Plague.' (Wellcome Library, London).

The Difeafes and Cafualties this Week.

Bortive	6	Kingfevil	10
Aged	54	Lethargy	1
oplexie	1	Murthered at Stepney	1
Iridden	1	Palfie	2
ncer	2	Plague	3880
ildbed	23	Plurifie	1
rifomes	15	Quinfie	6
llick	1	Rickets	23
nfumption	174	Rifing of the Lights	19
nvulfion	88	Rupture	2
opfie	40	Sciatica	1
owned 2, one at St. Kath-ower, and one at Lambeth	2	Scowring	13
ver	353	Scurvy	1
ula	1	Sore legge	1
x and Small-pox	10	Spotted Feaver and Purples	190
x	2	Starved at Nurfe	1
nd dead in the Street at Bartholomew the Lefs	1	Stilborn	8
		Stone	2
ghted	1	Stopping of the ftomach	16
ngrene	1	Strangury	1
wt	1	Suddenly	1
cf	1	Surfeit	87
ping in the Guts	74	Teeth	113
ndies	3	Thrufh	3
ofthume	18	Tiffick	6
nts	21	Ulcer	2
d by a fall down ftairs at , Thomas Apoftle	1	Vomiting	7
		Winde	8
		Wormes	18

Chriftned { Males — 83, Females — 83, In all — 166 }   Buried { Males — 2656, Females — 2663, In all — 5319 }   Plague — 3880

Increafed in the Burials this Week —————— 1289
Parifhes clear of the Plague ———— 34; Parifhes Infected ———— 96

Affize of Bread fet forth by Order of the Lord Maior and Court of Aldermen, A penny Wheaten Loaf to contain Nine Ounces and a half, and three half-penny White Loaves the like weight.

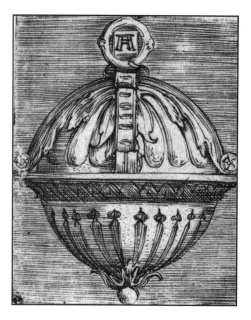

'Sixteenth-century pomander for protecting against the plague.' (Rijksmuseum, Netherlands)

'Two physicians, one representing George Thompson dissecting the corpse of a plague sufferer, from his book on the plague Loimotomia; or the Pest Anatomized, 1666.' (Wellcome Library, London)

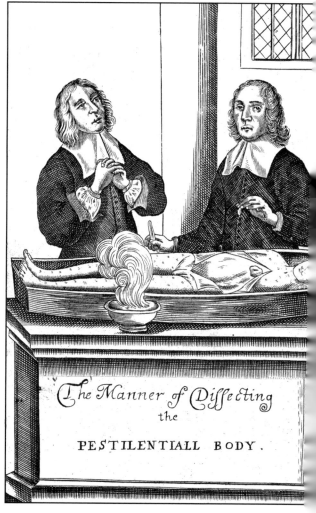

The Manner of Dissecting the

PESTILENTIALL BODY.

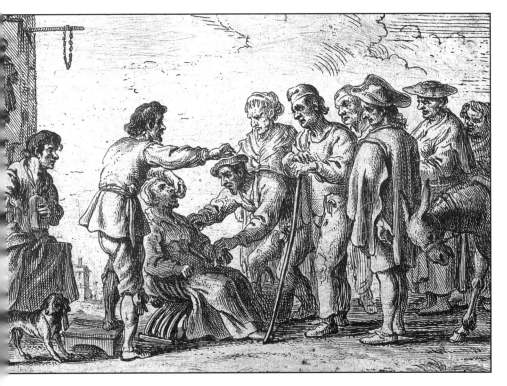

thache: 'A travelling healer demonstrating the extraction of a tooth from the mouth of a
man patient, before a crowd of onlookers.' (Wellcome Library, London)

ereal Disease: 'A man in bed suffering from syphilis, amidst a busy domestic scene, 1600.'
ellcome Library, London)

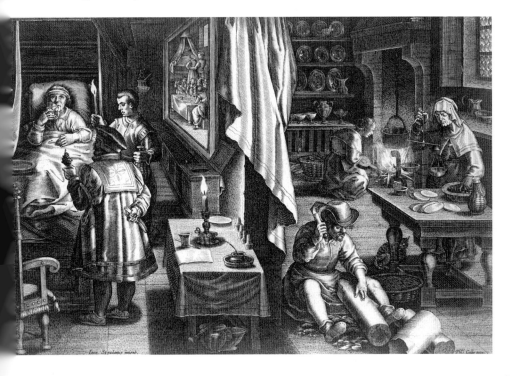

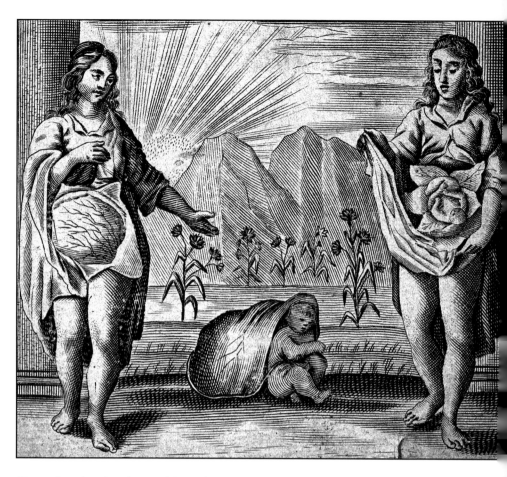

'Engraving showing the gravid womb and its blood supply on the left and a child in the womb on the right, 1676.' (Wellcome Library, London)

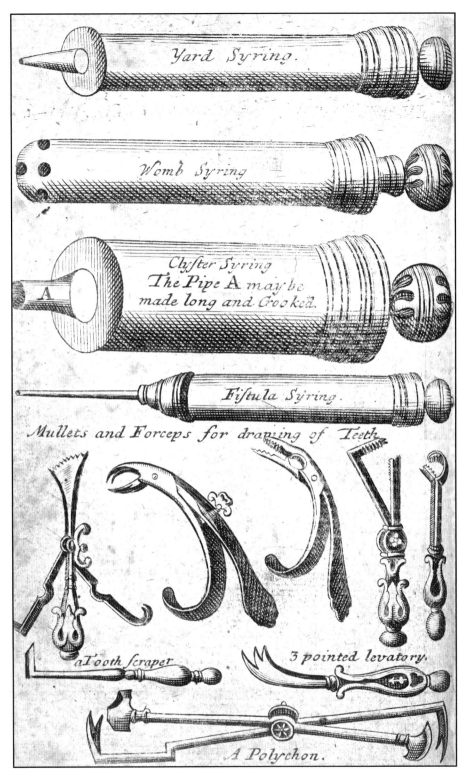

'Constipation was often relieved using a clyster or liquid enema delivered to the rectum via syringes such as these. Note the different types of syringes, for delivering internal medicines including ones for the penis, the vagina, and the rectum.' (Wellcome Library, London)

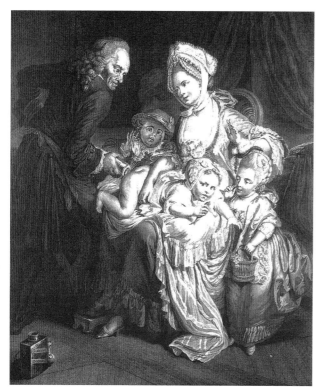

'A doctor administers a clyster to a greedy little boy who is laying across his mothers lap, his two siblings watch the scene with amusement.' (Wellcome Library, London)

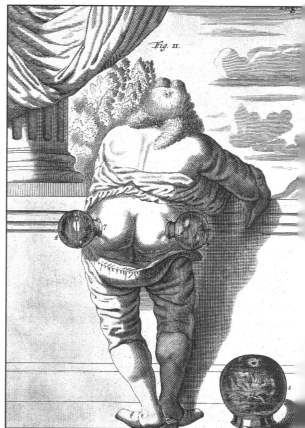

Cupping: 'Illustration showing the position of two cupping glasses on the buttocks of a gentleman, 1694.' (Wellcome Library, London)

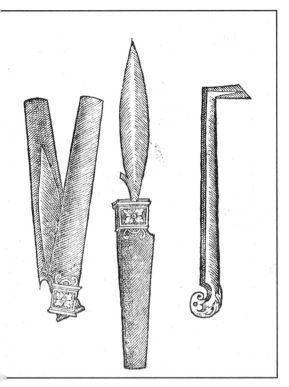

'"Lancets and flambets": Instruments for blood-letting, 1612.' (Wellcome Library, London)

'Ointment jar. With the name of Stewart, 12–13, Broad Street, Manufactory.' (Wellcome Library, London)

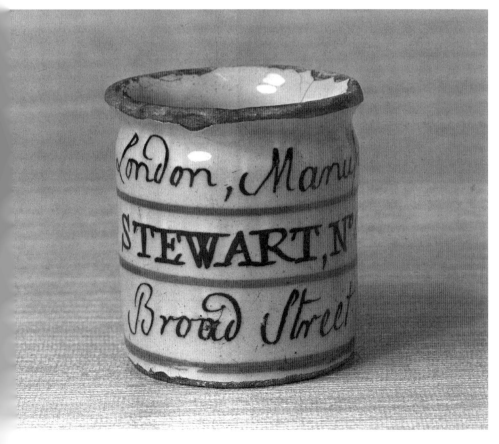

For a Rheum in the Eyes.

Take a handful of bitter Almonds, and let them lie in Elder berry-water 3 or 4 Days, untill they will blanch, then blanch them, and beat them with an Ounce of Spirit of Benjamin, and a handful of Raisins of the Sun stond, beat 'em alltogether, and so keep it in a Gallipot, and wash your hands or Face with it. It will dry away the Rheum in the Eyes.

For a Whitelow, or Fellon.

Lay to it New Cow Dung 2 or 3 Times a Day, it will draw & heal it.

For a pain in the Side.

Take 4 grains of Frankincence, and waste it in an Apple, and eat it when You go to Bed, for 4 Nights together.

For them that can't make Water

Take a head of Garlick and bruise it, and put the Juice it into half a pint of Ale and give it to drink, or you m— give it in White wine, and sweeten it with Syrup of Marsh Mallows.

'A page from Susan Tully, Lady Hoare's "Book of Receipts for Cookery and Pastry, etc", containing treatment on the following: 'For a Rheum in the Eyes', 'For a Whitelow or Fello— 'For a Pain in the Side' and 'For them that can't make Water'. Eighteenth Century. (Wellco— Library, London)

Chapter 12

Dropsy: Drowning in Water

'How doth a Dropsie melt him to a flood, / Making each vein run water more than blood?'

– Dr Henry King

According to William Sermon, who served in the parliamentary forces before setting up a fashionable London medical practice after the Restoration, 'the dropsy', or 'dropsie', was a condition characterised by 'a preternatural' accumulation of watery or windy humours in the body. Like jaundice, it was not always considered to be a disease in its own right, but could be a symptom in a range of disorders and, like gout, it had different names depending upon the part of the body afflicted and the type of humour that collected. As ascites it was a watery swelling of the belly, and sometimes the legs and feet. While a tympanites got 'its Name from a Drum, because the *Abdomen* is extended or stretched forth like to a Drum' with wind. Finally, if phlegmatic humours plagued the whole body the disorder was called an anasarca or a *leucophlegmatia* – because the swollen body appeared white. Sermon was well acquainted with the condition. In 1661 a patient suffering from the condition consulted him, and by the following year he had devised his own pill to treat the disease, which he successfully tried out on a friend.

Sermon explained that the disease was most often caused by a 'great coldness of the Liver', which meant that instead of producing good blood, it sent out 'raw and phlegmatic' humours. Several things could cause this to happen, including over-indulgence in small beer and cold water, the loss of too much blood or a long-standing ague, gout, or venereal disease. Sermon was keen to point out that a particular cause of the disease was the 'excessive drinking of Brandy, which beyond all other Liquors commonly drunk, Burns and dries up the Radical Moisture, hinders the circulation of the Blood, and turns it into a serous matter.' While Galenic practitioners focused on the liver, an English compilation of Jean Baptiste van Helmont's works showed that chemical physicians thought otherwise: 'I could never conceive, that the Liver should be the cause of the Dropsy [...] Wherefore the vice hath seemed to me, to subsist rather in the Kidney than in the Liver.'

He listed numerous examples of patients' bodies that, once dead of the disease, revealed that their livers were perfectly intact. Van Helmont's explanation concurs much more with modern thinking because, nowadays, medics and patients are aware that kidney disease, amongst other conditions, results in this type of swelling, although this can be connected to both liver and heart disease as well.

The association of dropsy with overindulgence, and particularly heavy drinking, could cause some confusion. The writer, gardener and diarist John Evelyn noted in his 'Kalendarium' that in October 1640 his father 'entered into a Dropsy, which was an indisposition, the most unsuspected, being a person so exemplarily temperate, and of admirable regiment.' Evelyn's father had already suffered bouts of ill health, but the dropsy he developed would be his last; Evelyn recorded sadly that on 24 December 1640 his father, 'that excellent man, and indulgent parent [...] departed this life'.

The symptoms of the disease included difficulty breathing and the body turning, according to Phillip Barrough, 'a naughty colour', a distaste for meat, and a great thirst, in addition to the obvious swelling. Troublingly, the prognosis for patients of this condition was not good. Many believed it to be an incurable, and sometimes fatal, disease. One observation corroborating this outcome recalled: 'In the Year 1658, we dissected a young Woman of four and twenty years of Age, which for seventeen years had laboured under that Distemper called *Ascites*, and at length died of it.' Isbrand van Diemerbroeck, the author, blamed the woman's lamentable condition on the fact that 'she had been cruelly used by her Parents, who were wont to kick and thump her', which had undermined and broken her lymphatic system. The patient described was very young to die from this disorder, but she was far from unusual. A Bill of Mortality for 1657 suggested that 631 people in the capital had died of the dropsy and tympany that year. Colonel Francis Lovelace, younger brother to the cavalier poet Richard, was the second governor of New York until the Dutch took back the territory, and he was sent home to London in disgrace. He was sent to the Tower of London for the dereliction of his duty in the colony. In April 1675 he was released on the grounds of ill health as he had developed dropsy; he died in December that year.

Dropsy was an uncomfortable and miserable chronic condition. The patient's swollen body limited their mobility, and left them short of breath. This could become quite extreme as an English translation of the work of renowned German Physician Daniel Sennert, for example, outlined: 'As the disease increases, the patient is forced continually to sit almost right up;

by reason of the great quantity of water oppressing the Diaphragm'. William Simpson recorded the case of Thomas Wested from Grimsby who was so swollen that he could not walk 20yds without a rest, so difficult was his breathing. This same author noted that in many respects those 'who die of *Dropsies* are (as we could easily show) really drowned' the same as 'happens by drowning in water.'

Perhaps due to the clear discomfort of sufferers medics of various kinds advocated a whole range of therapeutic regimes and surgical interventions designed to limit the progress of the disease or cure it altogether. Ancient and medieval practitioners had recorded the 'tapping' operation as a cure for the dropsy and their early modern counterparts followed suit. Van Diemerbroeck debated in his medical text the value of this procedure. It involved puncturing the navel with a curved needle attached to a thread to create a passage to disperse the accumulated watery humours trapped inside the abdomen. He noted that while stories circulated of patients cured in this way, it was best to follow nature. If the humours did not naturally seep out from the belly button to find release, then such an operation would be prejudicial to recovery. Other medics described 'tapping the abdomen', rather than the navel. An alternative was to lightly scarify or blister the legs, but again this had to be done carefully to avoid gangrene.

Although the disease was connected to the production of bad blood, removing this problematic fluid was not always considered a good idea. Arthur Jessop, a Yorkshire apothecary working in the mid-eighteenth century ended up embroiled in controversy when he bled a patient. He recorded in his diary that he had called on a Mr Kaye who requested to be bled. However, two days later on 23 June 1744, he followed up with the note that 'I hear that when Mrs Kaye came home on Thursday at night after I was come away she was very much displeased that Mr Kaye had been bled and said she would not have him bled for £20.' The disgruntled patient's wife called for a second opinion from a Mr Hardcastle, who reported that 'it was very bad thing to bleed Mr Kaye who was in danger of a Dropsy'. Perhaps feeling attacked or undermined, Jessop noted that 'I would loath have bled him and desired him to consider better of it, but he forced me to bleed him against my mind, and held the vessel himself [...] whether I would or no and he bled a very large quantity.' Despite the fact that Mr Kaye appeared to be better by 5 July, this episode evidently prayed on Jessop's mind as he recorded in several subsequent entries that he had enquired both about Mr Kaye's health and considered why there had been such uproar about the course of treatment. Mrs Kaye clearly did not forgive Jessop as he wrote in his diary that on 13 November he had visited Mr Kaye, but that Mrs Kaye 'was very angry and asked me if I was come to bleed Mr Kaye again and was in such a passion that she left the room and would not sit at Dinner with us.' Mr Kaye was in complete disagreement with his wife claiming that 'Hardcastle was a damnable liar, and his Physick made his legs to swell'. He argued that Jessop's ministrations had done him much good to alleviate his condition. Jessop concluded 'we parted very kindly and he thanked me for my visit.'

Goat's Dung and Child's Urine

Rather than letting blood, most commonly healers recommended pills, drinks and evacuating medicines designed to purge the body of these superfluous watery humours, or 'discutient' medicines – ones that dispersed wind from the body. One early eighteenth-century medical text recommended the roots of flower-de-luce and elaterium (the juice of a wild cucumber). Michael Ettmüller, a professor of botany and anatomy and eminent physician in Leipzig, the author of these recommendations, cautioned that care had to be taken to moderate the effects of these purges, because taking them too frequently could result in the body's 'laudable humours' being melted down and expelled with potentially damaging results. However, as with much medical advice in early modernity, others argued the contrary. John Locke recorded that only 'plentiful and repeated purging' would work as 'small ones only increase the disease'. Figuring out the appropriate level of purging in the midst of contrary advice was perhaps a precarious practice.

John Hall tended to be a conservative practitioner and used herbal cures over more invasive procedures wherever possible. So when Captain Francis Bassett saw the doctor for dropsy, which caused swollen feet, he treated the 50-year-old with emetic and laxative drugs. These gave 'seven vomits and three stools.' The next day, after more pills, Bassett had 'seven Stools and the next day one Pill gave five Stools, and with happy event, for thereby he could both better walk and breathe.' To maintain the recovery, Hall gave him a 'sweating Potion', which 'perfectly cured him.' Hall had evidently found the correct balance of purges.

Another of John Hall's patients needed repeated purges to cure her of a dropsy she developed after the birth of her third child. He treated Mrs Fiennes, who had a postnatal fever the third day after the delivery, with cooling cordials, but Hall felt this had been too much since she developed a swollen right thigh and leg. Her midwife had attempted a cure by applying a plaster of red lead and pressing it on very firmly, but when this didn't work she called in the doctor. Initially, Mrs Fiennes responded to Hall's purges, but after a couple of days described to him that she had felt like she was suffocating with phlegm in the night, much like the drowning sensation described by others. Her recovery was slow, but after a few days she was able to walk about with the aid of a 'staff'. Hall prescribed ten different treatments altogether, the last of which, to maintain the recovery, was a clyster given twice a week and was made from a child's urine as the principle ingredient. Eventually, she was 'restored to her former health.'

Away from the medics, purges were the remedy of choice in manuscript recipe collections as well. A book attributed to Mary Chantrell included 'an excellent remedy for the timpany or dropsy', made from five pints of Rhenish wine mixed with ashes made from broom (the plant genisteae, rather than the sweeping implement). Bridget Hydes's recipe book included a much more complex concoction made with two types of wine, horseradish, sweet fennel seeds and roots, winter savory, sweet marjoram, watercress, nettles, and water. Thankfully, it was noted that it was available 'ready made at every Apothecaries shop.'

If the disease progressed to an anasarca, Michael Ettmüller suggested that volatile preparations of tartar and the volatile salt of hartshorn might be useful. However, an important caveat noted that: 'Man's Urine, or that of Sheep is very effectual among poor People', as well as 'Goose dung given to a dram in distilled Urine.' The remedies suggested continued in this rather unpalatable (to modern readers) vein, including 'Earthworms putrefied with Moss of Earth, and baken with Dough in an Oven, given to a spoonful twice a day; the Powder of dried Toads, the Heads and Entrails being thrown away [and] the Powder of greasy Beetles, or of Hog-lice.' To aid the removal of wind, people might apply aromatics to the soles of the feet, belly and cods (testicles). These included the leaves of greater celandine, quilted bags containing aromatic seeds and bran, human excrement, goat or horse dung boiled in mint water, or mixed with human urine made into a cataplasm, or a cataplasm made from bruised cockles and goat dung.

It is clear that the kinds of oedemas represented under the catchall diagnosis of dropsy were from many and various causes. Whereas now investigations would look to find the cause of the swelling as much as to relieve the symptoms, in early modernity it was considered a worrying condition, for which purging the body of corrupt humours, by a variety of means, was thought best.

Chapter 13

Gout: A Painful Guest

'The knotty Gout doth sadly torture me'
– Anne Bradstreet

Gout, like venereal disease, is almost synonymous with the early modern era and particularly the eighteenth century when, some scholars have claimed, the disease appeared to reach epidemic proportions, fostered by the rise of consumer society, increased affluence and leisure time. Yet it is a disease with a long pedigree. Hippocratic writers knew about the disease and Roman authors suggested that the early days of the Republic were marked by the rarity of the condition while the spread of luxury under the Empire caused a resurgence. However, when these authors spoke of gout they were actually describing a range of arthritic conditions. Thomas Harper's 1633 *Gutta Podagrica* explained that: 'Generally, all such aches as are incident to any joint, we call the *Gout*'. Through until early modernity these conditions were differentiated according to the body part they affected. Thus, Harper noted, when it fell upon the feet it was known as *podagra*, in the fingers it was *chiragra*, in the hips *sciatica*, and in the knees *gonagra*. The word 'gout' comes from the Greek for rheumatism, which in Latin became *gutta*, or drop, which in French became *goutte* and in English gout.

In the eighteenth century, as the disease became much more prevalent, the use of the terms *chiragra* and *gonagra* diminished, and 'the Gout' was increasingly distinguished as a particular disease afflicting gentlemen. As William Stukeley claimed in 1736 ''tis nonsense to divide it into *podagra, chiragra, mentagra, gonagra, talia,* and the like ridiculous names, as if it were not terrible enough, unless split into 100 terrors.' Physicians also increasingly spoke of 'irregular gout', which rebounded from the joints into the major organs – the liver, heart, and brain, and the 'flying gout', where the pains skipped around the body at random.

Gout and the Spider

Despite the eighteenth-century focus on social rank, gout throughout this era was associated with luxury and the upper classes. Many medical writers explained who was likely to be afflicted with the disease by reciting a particular story about the gout and a spider. The anonymously authored *Poorman's Plaster Box* (1634) related the story in all its glory to show that the rich and the idle were most likely to suffer from the disease:

'A tale that is true enough'

A great while ago, when Monsieur Gout was not so rich (as now he is), he was forced to travel, as other poor men are sometime, in his travel he met with a spider, whose journey lay as Mr Gout's did: they being both benighted they sought lodging, and came to a poor man's house, which the Gout took up for his lodging, for he being always a lazy companion, would go no farther, but the Spider being more nimble, went to a rich man's house, and there took up his lodging for that night.

The next day they met again, and asked each other of their entertainment the past night, mine said the Gout was the worst as ever I had, for I had no sooner touched the poor man's legs, thinking there to take my rest, but up he gets, and to threshing he goes, so that I had no rest the whole night. And I, said the Spider, had no sooner begun to build my house, in the rich man's chamber, but the Maid came with a broom, and tore down all my work, and so fiercely did pursue me, that I had so much ado to save my life, as ever I had.

Seeing it is so then, said the Gout, we will change lodging, I will go to the rich man's house, and thou shalt go to the poor man's: they both were well content, and did so and found such ease and rest in their lodging, that they resolved never to remove, for the Spider built and was not troubled, the Gout he was entertained with a soft cushion, with down Pillows, with dainty Caudles, and delicate broths; in brief: he did like it so well that ever since he takes up his lodging with rich men, where I desire that he should take his rest, rather than in my poor house.

The author concluded that gout 'commonly keeps good company, as Bishops, Cardinals, Dukes, Earls, Lords, Knights, Judges, Gentlemen, and Merchants', as these men were more likely to indulge in luxury. John Peachi's *Some Observations made upon the Calumba wood* (1694) also suggested that it was most likely to affect those in the public realm. He claimed that 'it falls generally upon Persons engaged in Public Affairs, upon whose Thought and Care the Service of their Country very much depends; and therefore [...] whoever proposes a way of Curing and Preventing it, would do great Service to States and Kingdoms, as well as to private Persons.'

What underpinned these claims was the knowledge that men and women who ate too much rich food and drank too much wine were more likely to develop gout. Whereas, medical theory suggested, the hard working poor, who lived on a frugal diet and who exercised regularly, were unlikely to develop these problems.

Medical theory, despite the existence of the disease in women, also argued that women were less likely to develop the disease because their bodies were better suited to regulating excess humours in the body, through menstruation, particularly those humours built up by a sedentary life. Men, however, were 'designed for action' and were, therefore, unsuited to regulating their bodies when excess was combined with a lack of exercise. Such theories were not born out in reality. Lady Joan Barrington evidently suffered a lameness brought on by gout and received letters from her daughter, Lady Mary Gerard, offering to send her 'oil of Exeter', as it was 'very good for the gout as I hear'.

The *Poorman's Plaster Box* explained that a rich diet produced 'crudities' in the body and an excess of humours, which were not dispersed appropriately because of the idleness of the wealthy. These excess humours dropped into the joints of the hands, feet, and knees (and occasionally other body parts), where they crystallised and hardened causing the joints to seize up. As Nicholas Culpeper's translation of Daniel Sennert's earlier works, which he called *Two Treatises* (1660), argued, there was little consensus about which humour in particular was the culprit. Some thought the humour was phlegm, others choler, others phlegm and choler, while yet others asserted it was phlegm mingled with blood, or a crude watery blood. What most authors did agree on was that the humour that fell onto the joints was salty and sharp, and thus caused pain. As we have seen, these causes mirror those of the stone – an inability of the body and stomach to adequately digest and 'use' all of the matter consumed leading to the build-up of calcareous matter. This did not go unnoticed by some commentators on the disease who argued that they were in fact the same disease, only differing in their position in the body.

It was evident to most commentators that certain foods and drinks, most notably wine, generated a 'tartarous' matter within the body and so were the most likely to contribute to the gout. At particular fault, *Two Treatises* claimed, were the wines produced in Austria, Hungary or Bohemia because the soil the grapes were grown in was 'fat, muddy, clayish, stony, and hath in it a Mineral' component. The rise in gout in the eighteenth century has also been linked to the Methuen Treaty with Portugal (1703), which dramatically increased the amount of port and fortified wine flowing into Britain.

But wine was not the only food to be criticised, some writers also claimed that capons, fish, eels, and cheese, could all provoke the disease.

Another more surprising factor thought to cause gout was excessive sexual activity. Johannes Groenvelt explained in 1697 that the 'violent motion' of venery (intercourse) triggered an excessive production of serum, which he considered to be the offending humour. Groenvelt claimed that '*immoderate Venus*' was in fact the most 'dangerous and hurtful' cause of gout. Earlier, Philemon Holland had also claimed that sex was a cause of the gout because it debilitated and cooled the body, thereby reducing its ability to disperse the humours. Gout was, then, a condition associated with the undesirable characteristics of gluttony, idleness and lasciviousness. It is perhaps little wonder that medical writers also offered the suggestion that the disease could be hereditary, thus explaining its presence in even the most upstanding of citizens. As George Philips wrote in an open letter to Sir John Gordon in 1691:

> *and tho it be ordinary to impute the Assaults of it to Excess in Diet, and other inordinate Pleasures; yet having in my Observations remarked how many Men and Women of the strictest Temperance, and singularly abstemious, have been in the most miserable manner afflicted with it, while others, setting no Limits to their Appetite, have for many Years indulged themselves in Excess, yet never suffered in any Symptoms of it.*

Indeed, William Stukeley, author of a pamphlet on gout published in 1734, and seller of a treatment based on the use of hot oils, claimed that his own gout was hereditary, perhaps to avoid the suggestion that he lacked self-control. Those who inherited a gouty disposition were not necessarily doomed to develop the disease, and were told that it could be avoided if strict regulation of the diet was implemented and adhered to.

An Irksome and Painful Guest

The disease was notoriously painful and debilitating. Even in its mildest forms, William Stukeley described it as an 'irksome guest'. More commonly it was said of patients that: 'They that feel it, know them too sensibly, and compare them to the gnawing of a dog, and to whatever is most direful and torturing.' Pepys recorded in his diary on 23 October 1662 that he had been to visit Sir William Penn, a naval officer, who was 'in great pain of the gout and in bed, [because he] cannot stir hand nor foot but with great pain.' Leaving his bedchamber to conduct business or social matters was evidently not a possibility for Penn, who received Pepys in his chamber or house several times because of his gout. Eventually Pepys reported that Penn had acquired, from Lady Lambert, a 'great chair, made on purpose for persons sick of that disease, for their ease.' By the late eighteenth century the pain of the gout was so well known that it was being represented visually as a devil or imp that bit, stabbed and burned the feet, as in the famous James Gillray etching. Such agonising illness of course could have rather undesirable affects and Lady Mary Rich, the Countess of Warwick, had to endure her husband's gout-induced irritability, which led him to forbid anyone from touching him or speaking to him.

Perhaps most disconcertingly, the pain of the disease was, for some, seasonal or periodic, returning at particular times of the year, or during particular bouts of weather, or following particular actions. John Pechey explained in *A Collection of Chronical Diseases* that the disease was liable to recur 'about the latter end of *January*, or the beginning of *February*.' There was thus some relief from the condition, but with the knowledge that it would return in the fullness of time. Stukeley noted that each bout of the illness debilitated the body further and was a little more severe: 'when they begin to return frequently, so incapacitate our limbs for action and necessary exercise, that the health and habit of the body and constitution suffer extremely and grow every year worse and worse.'

A Friend in Disguise

Despite the dire situation of gouty patients, some medical commentators were keen to point out that in old age, gout could actually be beneficial. In *A Problem Concerning the Gout* George Philips claimed that if the 'Indications of it do commence in his declining Age' a man should not use means to repel it, 'but patiently to endure the Fit, as a lucky, though sharp Composition for more fatal Maladies.' How the gout prevented more serious conditions the author didn't elucidate, but rather suggested that Englishmen look to their continental counterparts to see how they should behave: 'I have heard or read of a Custom used in the *Low-Countries*, That when a Man after Fifty falls into the *Gout*, his Friends come about him, they make a Feast, and rejoice at this hopeful prolongation of Life, and a probable addition of Twenty or Thirty years to it.'

Peruvian Bark and other Remedies

Pains in the joints of the hands and feet, particularly when stretching, a painful weariness, catarrhs, wandering pains in the limbs, and a heaviness of the head, combined with an inability to move, heralded the onset of a fit of the gout. This was soon followed by a swelling and reddening of the afflicted joints.

Treatments for the gout included both internal remedies and topical applications. As John Marten noted in his amusingly named text, *Attila of the Gout* (1713) there were a plethora of suggestions offered to patients as 'every one almost having his particular Remedy.' Many were intended to counter the perceived cause of the disease: poor digestion. John Locke, for example, argued that because it was a 'disease of malnutrition', Peruvian bark would 'help the digestion and assimilation of the food' and so ease the condition. Other remedies applied early in the flare-up, according to Groenevelt, were intended to drive the humour out of the afflicted joint. These, often cooling and astringent medicines, were a risky strategy though because they might push the humour into another joint, or towards more 'noble' (important) organs. If the humour couldn't be 'repulsed' from the joints, then it had to be evacuated by sweating or vomits.

Many practitioners offered their own particular suggestions for a cure; William Stukeley advocated a treatment based on the application of a particular hot oil that he 'persuaded the preparer' to send to him in London. John Peachi meanwhile advocated the use of Calumba wood taken in a variety of ways, and recited anecdotes from happy customers to show its efficacy. These included a young merchant who had been attending the baths without relief, a young gentlewoman who had been to the hot-houses, a gouty old man who was confined to his bed, and a 50-year-old gentlewoman who had been undergoing phlebotomy – although, of course, all these testimonial cases might have been invented to help sales.

There were also some rather more gruesome cures offered for the gout. *The Secrets of Maister Alexis of Piemont* (1568) suggested that the patient take the skin from the heels of a vulture; the skin from the right foot was to be laid on the right foot of the patient, and likewise with the left foot. The author claimed that the patient would see that 'in half an hour the pain will go away. Which is a marvellous thing.' Puppies were thought to have a particular virtue in appeasing the pain of the gout and so various plasters suggested in medical texts such as *Choice and Rare Experimented Receipts in Physick and Chirurgery* (1675) included the 'grease' (fat) of a 'puppy-dog'. If this was too complex, Thomas Lupton's *Thousand Notable Things* (1579) advocated taking a 'whelp' 'especially of one colour', which had been 'cloven in two parts through the midst of the back', and laying this to the afflicted joints. He claimed that 'this I know to be an excellent thing.' Likewise, John Marten recorded that Petrus Borellus had advised patients 'to let young puppies lie with him: For, says he, they'll contract the Distemper, and the Patient will be wonderfully relieved.'

As William Stukeley argued though, it was not in the power of any remedy to overcome the gout in those who would not confine themselves to a sober lifestyle and the use of exercise. Patients were therefore strongly advised to regulate their diet and activities.

Opening the Skin: Surgical Cures

If remedies didn't work and gout afflicted someone for a long time, medical writers warned that the sharp humours that had collected in the joints would begin to harden much like in the stone. These hard concretions were difficult to disperse and might require surgical intervention. This was a relatively minor surgical procedure, compared to amputation or couching for cataracts; a small incision was made in the skin of the hands or feet to allow the stones to be removed. *Two Treatises* explained the different outcomes of this action:

> *if the Skin be opened, out there runneth a matter, sometimes fluid and white, and sometimes like unto Plaster or white Lime; and sometimes the matter is hard, like unto gravelly stones that may be crumbled.*

Operations to ease the gout were just as liable as any others to fail and it has been noted that the politician Roger Boyle, first earl of Orrery, composed devotional poems towards the end of his life, having been incapacitated by a botched operation meant to ease his condition.

For those suffering from the gout, the search for analgesics and cures was a long one, and often such measures brought little relief. As Sir Thomas Baines wrote to Lady Anne Conway 'I [have been] nailed to my bed for these five weeks by the Gout', typifying the pain patients felt. Physician and sufferer Thomas Sydenham concurred that there was no cure and that pain relief was rarely effective. He lamented that many people tried to offer cures but that 'the excellent art of medicine should be so much disgraced by such trifles, with which the credulous are deceived, either through the ignorance or knavery' of the sellers. Gout, for many, was a seasonal trial to be endured, not cured; one that incapacitated and immobilised.

Chapter 14

Irritating Infestations: Rubbing and Scratching

'Mark but this flea, and mark in this, I
How little that which thou deniest me is'

– John Donne

E arly modern life was rife with creepy crawlies, many of which, people reported, infested the body and caused ill health and disease. From worms to lice, men and women were quite accustomed to dealing with home and bodily invasion. Samuel Pepys recorded in his diary that his wife removed lice from his body as a part of his personal hygiene routine:

So to my wife's chamber, and there supped and got her [to] *cut my hair and look* [at] *my shirt, for I have itched mightily these six or seven days; and when all came to all, she finds that I am louzy, having found in my head and body above 20 lice, little and great; which I wonder at, being more than I have had I believe almost these 20 years.*

More than this, the invention of the microscope in this era meant that, for the first time, people could clearly see these bodily invaders. Robert Hooke's famous study *Micrographia*, published in 1665, included detailed drawings of mites and fleas, made possible by viewing them microscopically. When he bought his copy, Pepys recorded that it was 'a most excellent piece, and of which I am very proud.' He later called it: 'The most ingenious book that ever I read in my life.' The use of the microscope offered exciting possibilities, as was made clear in a 1660s advertisement for a book of directions to accompany the 'Famous Medicines' *Pulvis Benedictus*, which noted that the book now came with a 'Historical Account of Worms', and experiments for their cure 'proved by that Admirable Invention of the Microscope'. The advert featured an image showing a selection of worms found in the body, presumably underlining the use of the microscope.

Although people were used to infestations, and some intellectuals found these microscopic creatures fascinating to study, people did not simply accept their presence. Many took active measures to clear their body of unwanted visitors. Samuel Hartlib recorded in his ephemerides for 1643 that perfuming the body with the smoke of quicksilver killed lice. He noted that this remedy was '*Probatum*' (proven), suggesting that he, or someone he knew, had put this method to good use. In 1656 he likewise recorded that oil of turpentine drove away all fleas, lice, and other vermin, and that when rubbed on a child's stomach it forced worms out of their bodies by vomiting or by stool.

Marks of Morality

These little invaders carried social and moral implications. Although they were believed to be the result of putrid heat in the body, augmented by eating 'Meats of thin juice', and in particular the consumption of figs, all lice, James Cooke claimed, 'breed in unclean Bodies, [and] filthy Garments'. They could also be caught from sharing 'unclean Beds with Lousie persons'. Implicitly then, having lice suggested a failing in personal hygiene, or a lack of discernment in choosing one's companions, which perhaps explains Pepys's surprised indignation at his wife having found twenty lice on his body. The historian Lisa T. Sarasohn has discovered that lousy people were often not considered as a separate entity from the vermin that lived on their bodies. Instead, they were considered to be accomplices and equally as worthy of disgust. In *A Treatise of Diseases Incident to the Skin* (1723), Daniel Turner's descriptions of the different kinds of lice explained that there was a specific sort found 'upon the foul Cloths, either Linen or Woollen of common Beggars, Jail-Birds and others', suggesting that these in particular carried connotations of beggarliness and social immorality. Lice didn't just threaten individual morality; their invasion of bodily space was also seen as a metaphor for the disintegration of the body politic during the civil war era. Their ability to afflict anyone of high or low status meant they represented subversion of authority – they were a kind of levelling agent in early modernity. In the Bible, lice were the fourth plague sent against the Egyptians when the Pharaoh refused to let the Israelites go. Lice were a scourge of God sent against the ungodly.

Sex and Insects

In his mock encomium on the louse, *Laus pediculi: An Apologetical Speech* (translated into English in 1634), Daniel Heinsius playfully praised the louse as subject to man's cruel oppressions in constantly trying to eradicate it. He emphasised that lice provide an opportunity to scratch a libidinous itch. He wrote: 'Often I have seen with what expressive delight, you use to rub and scratch, sometimes your head, sometimes your sides, sometimes another part, to which this guest gives the gentle itching twist.' The sexual connotations of this itching are clear, but Heinsius also made a less than subtle hint at a more deviant masturbatory pleasure that lice facilitated, when he called it 'your so mighty fricative pleasure'. The intimate relationship between a person and their parasites was also used to poetic effect by the English poet John Donne in 'The Flea', published posthumously in 1633. The poet attempts to woo a mistress by arguing that since the flea has bitten both lovers, then their bloods are already intermingled:

> And in this flea, our two bloods mingled be;
> Thou know'st that this cannot be said
> A sin, nor shame nor loss of maidenhead,

Therefore, since they are already joined inside the flea, it cannot be a sin to have sex. Unfortunately for the speaker, his mistress, 'Cruel and sudden, hast thou since /Purpled thy nail, in blood of innocence?', killed the flea and quashed his argument.

In William Shakespeare's *King Lear* (1608), the fool's riddle suggested that: 'He that has a house to put his head in, has a good headpiece, the Codpiece that will house before the head, has any the head and he shall louse', suggesting that foolish men, led by their genitals, would be liable to catching pubic lice or crabs, the existence of which exercised medical writers too. A new edition of James Cooke's *Mellificium Chirurgiæ* in 1717 stated: 'Those called Crab-lice that are flat and broad, grow under the Arm-pits, Eye-brows, near and on the privy Parts.' Daniel Turner wrote that these were particularly difficult to dislodge, but Cooke recommended an unguent containing mercury and sulphur, which he said was 'excellent' for the purpose. Clearly not everyone was familiar with this cure, as Turner recorded treating a young man who had suffered from 'troublesome' itching of this nature. The patient had taken the drastic measure of having 'clipt off' all his pubic hair, and when Turner revealed that his plight was the result of lice, it was 'found he was an utter Stranger, having never heard of them before.'

Diseases and Lice

Lice were not simply annoyances; they could cause serious health problems. Daniel Turner's early eighteenth-century treatise on skin complaints told readers:

That not only Worms of sundry Kinds, but also other living Creatures are found therein (however they come there) is too notorious to want Proof: Nay that our Blood is full of them, that most of our Diseases take Rise from them, more especially the Cancer, Itch, Ring-worm, &c.

Even when unconnected to these more virulent disorders, lice posed a significant threat. Turner warned that: 'It is recorded by Authors both ancient and modern, that diverse Persons have come to their Ends being devoured of Lice'. Perhaps more worryingly, Turner suggested that in cases where medicine had not been applied to the body, a sudden abandonment of a body by these 'filthy Vermin' was 'reckoned to prognosticate Death or speedy Mortality'.

Worms of Different Types

Lice might have caused itching and uncomfortable skin conditions, but worms invaded the internal organs of the body, often bringing greater sickness. Worms were a familiar problem both inside and outside of the body. Samuel Pepys recorded in his diary that on 26 June 1662, he had come home with Commissioner Pett for dinner 'where my stomach was turned when my sturgeon came to table, upon which I saw very many little worms creeping, which I suppose was through the staleness of the pickle.' That his servants had served up such a meal is worrying, and evidently Pepys was less than *au fait* with his food being infested.

Worms were particularly associated with children's bodies. J.S., the author of *Paidon Nosemata*, attributed this to the weakness of children's stomachs and their diets. He claimed that:

Worms are very familiar to Children, by reason of crudity and corrupt Phlegm, from their eating of fruits and milk after other meats, for it is observed that sucking [breast feeding] Children which eat Flesh are most troubled with Worms because their tender Stomach cannot concoct solid meat, and therefore it corrupts and breeds Worms.

He also noted that there were many different types of worms that bred in the human body, he described these by their shape: 'broad and long', or 'small', and by their colour: red, ash-coloured, yellow, or white.

The signs that a child was sick with worms were: a swollen belly, bad breath, difficulty sleeping, trembling, grinding the teeth, rubbing the nose, paleness, dark and hollow eyes, and the spitting of much phlegm. Yet it was acknowledged that different worms would produce different symptoms. For example, 'broad' worms that appeared in a child's excrement caused an insatiable appetite.

The prognosis also changed depending upon the type of worm in the body. Small worms were easier to expel because they bred in the bowels, where medicines could be applied, meaning a patient was more likely to recover; while broad worms were most hurtful to the body because they remained in the body a long time. The posthumous English translation of Franciscus Sylvius's *Of Children's Diseases* (1675) warned that the '*long and smooth*' worms that afflicted all children could be very dangerous, consuming the body, causing fever, falling-sickness (epilepsy) or even death.

De-worming

As with most diseases in this era, the fundamental of curing worms was to amend the diet to prevent the build-up of crudities and corruption in the stomach. *Of Children's Diseases* (1675) recommended that children were given bread with their meat because it would stop them over-consuming meat – the cause of the worms – by sooner filling them up. Certain sweet foods that were more liable to cause worms were also to be avoided, including sweet milk, cheese, and green fruit (particularly plums). Despite this advice, a remedy recorded in Mary Chantrell's recipe book was a mixture of milk, wormwood, rue, and lavender sweetened with honey.

In addition to amending a child's diet, purges and other medicines were used to try and hasten the expulsion of the worms through the body's natural passages. These purges were moderated according to the age and constitution of the child. Older children could be given the stronger, and also more bitter, remedies like aloes, *hiera picra* (a mixture of canella bark and honey), and rhubarb. Robert Pemell, whose 1653 book declared he was a 'Practitioner in *Physick*, at *Cranebrooke* in *Kent*', advised that bitter things should be administered by the mouth and sweet things in clysters, because as the worms moved to feed on the sweet remedies, they would be drawn towards the fundament. John Hall was perhaps following this advice when he treated Talbot, the Countess of Salisbury's first child, for worms and a fever when he was a year old. He injected a clyster (a liquid enema) of milk and sugar to provoke defecation. This was apparently successful and the child voided four worms. To follow up, he gave a julep (a sweet flavoured drink made of sugar syrup) of burnt hartshorn, and a poultice made of spiders webs and nutshells. The boy recovered in three days and Hall noted that the Countess rewarded him greatly.

Samuel Hartlib suggested that the problem could also be the solution. He noted in his ephemerides (his journal) for 1634 that although burnt harts-horn was a good remedy, the best was 'to take one of the greatest worms which does come from a child wash it clean dry it then pulverize it give of that powder a certain quantity.' In another note he suggested that: 'Earth worms put alive into a linen bag' and hung from either the navel or stomach when the child went to bed would provide a cure. Having said this, in 1654 he recorded that: 'the only remedy against worms was a herb called French Pinget.' He claimed: 'There is such an antipathy between it and them that they are presently voided by stool or vomit.' This was evident, Hartlib declared, as an author who had written a book on this subject explained that six of his own children had died of worms, but the rest were preserved by the use of the herb.

As with many of the diseases explored in this book, John Peachi published a pamphlet advocating the supposedly wondrous effects of an exotic medicine for the worms in 1695. The 'Mexico Seeds', he claimed, power-fully expelled worms from the bodies of men, women and children, as well as resisting the putrefaction of the humours. One advantage of this cure was that whereas: 'Many young Children have been destroyed by Worms, because they would not take bitter unpleasant Medicines; but this being given only in Drops, and insensibly proved very successful towards the Preservation of their Lives.' Other medical practitioners were also aware that the bitter medicines required in treating this disease were unpalatable to children and so should be adapted. Isbrand van Diemerbroeck added syrup of lemons to the quicksilver remedy he prescribed for the 6-year-old son of Mr Cooper because the child was 'averse to all manner of Physick.' Hannah Newton's 2012 study of childhood ailments has found that adapting remedies for chil-dren's sweeter tooth was a relatively common practice, and was certainly not restricted to the treatment of worms.

Creeping Forth at the Mouth and Nostrils

As we have seen here, many remedies aimed to encourage worms to move through the digestive tract and leave the body. However, worms were thought to move around inside the body and find numerous exits. Felix Platter's *Golden Practice of Physick* (1664) described one patient who was suffering from colic who 'made Urine with infinite small worms like mites in cheese, swimming alive therein; which dying, sank down in a great lump to the bottom.' While *The Secret Miracles of Nature* (1658) reported that:

> *It hath been seen sometimes miraculously, that long and round Worms especially, have scrambled upwards, and crept forth at the mouth and the nostrils: and they do this by an inbred natural motion, if a man be long fasting. For then they bite the stomach, and seek for meet, and when they find none to satisfy them and preserve their lives, they creep upwards, and hunt for meat as far as the very throat. For they by their natural instinct perceive, that the food comes in that way, and the nostrils being open to the very throat almost, they creep thither, and tickle the part, or else they are cast forth by sneezing, or are pulled forth with ones forefingers.*

John Hall also reported an occurrence like this. Richard Wilmore of Norton, aged 14, vomited several black worms that had red heads and six feet and were an inch and a half long. Hall noted that they 'crept like Earwigs'. Another child, aged 3, had four dead worms pulled from a tumour on his stomach, while five crawled out, still living. John Evelyn recorded in his diary that on 9 August 1682, he had attended the Royal Society, a learned society for the advancement of science formed in 1660, and given royal backing in 1663. The Society was attended by the great and good, to hear lectures and watch demonstrations of experiments. On this day, a Dr Tyson showed the audience a 24ft worm 'voided' by one of his patients. The poor man, it was said, had 'endured such torment in his bowels, that he thought of killing himself.' The ejection of a worm of that length could hardly have been much more unpleasant.

As these accounts show, dealing with insects, worms, and other parasites, was a part of daily life in early modernity. Inconvenient and annoying at best, they could also carry other diseases, and bites could become infected, which was significantly more dangerous in the pre-antibiotic era. Little wonder then that authors of medical texts wrote so much on these creatures.

Chapter 15

Pestilential Plague: A Divine Affliction

'mirth is both physical and wholesome against the plague'
– Thomas Dekker

During the Great Plague of 1665 an anonymous author wrote that, 'Of all the diseases whereunto the body of man is subject, the Plague or Pestilence is the most terrible and fearful, and most contagious therefore we must seek all means, both Natural and Artificial, to preserve our selves and Families from it.' The author did not exaggerate. Writing at the time of the great plague, many believed that God was punishing England for the sins and chaos of the civil war era. Plague was one of the three punishments God imposed on the sinful populace along with war and famine, and it occurred at intervals seemingly at least once every generation. The plague was referred to as 'the pestilance' colloquially, often shortened to 'the pest' from the French *peste*. The name plague is a Latin borrowing from *plāga* meaning affliction or illness especially, as in this case, one thought to be a divine punishment. The Great Plague of 1665, like the 1603 outbreak in which 30,000 Londoners died, was a devastating one, the latest in a series of outbreaks stretching back to medieval times. The deaths were frequent, and the plague struck quickly and hard, patients could die within a matter of days and medical practitioners seemed impotent to cure it.

In one way bubonic plague was a recognisable disease. As the author of *The Plagues Approved Physician* noted 'The surest token of all to know the infected of the plague, is, if there do arise and engender botches behind the ears, or under the arm holes.' Beyond this though the disease was rather complex, encompassing a range of symptoms that may, or may not, appear in every case making it much more difficult to identify. The same author's overview of the disease's symptoms highlighted that they were akin to those of many other diseases:

First when the outward members are cold, and the inward parts burning hot, when there is a pain and heaviness of the head, and a great inclination to sleep. A weariness, heaviness, and difficulty in breathing. A sadness and carefulness of the mind: a change of countenance, with a frowning look of the eyes: loss of stomach and appetite: immoderate

thirst and often vomiting: a bitterness and dryness of the mouth: The
pulse frequent, small and deep, the Urine troublous [sic], *thick, and*
stinking like beasts' urine.

Plague could occur at any time of the year but was seasonal in that it was
more prevalent and virulent in the summer months. The Stuart monarchs
were well aware of this and would limit their ceremonies for healing the
King's Evil by the divine touch at these times, in order to limit the king's
exposure to infectious people.

Religious Responses

As mentioned above, plague was widely seen as a divine punishment for sin. After
the Reformation one interpretation was that God was expressing his anger that
Roman Catholics were tolerated in England. In the Great Plague of 1665 many
people attributed the punishment to the diseased body politic, which had been
cut off from its head by the regicide in 1649, and so needed to be purged and
restored. Given that sin was the cause of the disease, it made logical sense that a
religious response was called for. In 1636 the government ordered that *A Form of
Common Prayer Together with an order for Fasting* should be printed and distributed amongst the populace. In 1640 they followed this up with a proclamation that
a fast should be observed throughout the realm. Both measures were intended to
heighten national piety and thereby diminish the effects of the plague.

These religious responses blended seamlessly with medical responses. As
we have already seen, prayer was an important part of healing throughout the
early modern period. The author of *The Plagues Approved Physician*, which
opened this chapter, included a range of medical prescriptions to combat
the disease. This pamphlet ended, though, with 'A Godly PRAYER, to be
used in the time of any common Plague or Sickness.' The prayer acknowledged that the depraved state of man had caused the plague: 'O Almighty
God, we do confess and acknowledge, that by many and diverse sins, we
have often and grievously offended thee, and therefore deserve most heavy
Plagues and punishments.' The prayer finished by beseeching God's mercy,
in this instance, in the guise of blessing 'all means which thou in mercy has
ordained for the preservation and cure of soul or body.'

Such religious responses were particularly crucial in this disease because
people died suddenly, and stories circulated of people who dropped dead in
the street. The prospect of a sudden death was alarming in terms of religious
beliefs, as it meant there was no time to properly prepare one's soul.

Searching the Dead and Shutting Up Houses

During times of plague the authorities attempted to limit the spread of the disease. In 1583 a set of twenty-one orders was published which became the standard response for combating outbreaks. These orders were published and republished as pamphlets in successive outbreaks. Although it is difficult to assess whether these printed orders were widely implemented, they do help us to understand 'official' responses to the plague. These *Orders* reveal that those in power believed that certain groups of people and certain behaviours were particularly responsible for the spread of disease. Measures to control the spread of infection therefore served a secondary function to improve the general morality and behaviour of the populace. The *Orders* printed in the seventeenth century devoted a whole section to 'loose Persons and idle Assemblies'. They suggested that 'no wandering Beggar [should] be suffered in the Streets of this City, in any fashion or manner whatsoever.' This would seem logical, preventing unknown people moving from place to place, potentially carrying the disease with them and introducing it to new areas. But the authors showed that this was a measure designed to tackle a pre-existing bug-bear: 'Forasmuch as nothing is more complained of, then the multitude of Rogues and wandering Beggars that swarm in every place about the City.'

In addition to removing beggars from the streets, the authorities also 'utterly prohibited' plays, bear-baiting, games, singing of ballads, feasts, dinners in taverns, and other activities that would cause groups of people to gather in one place. Alehouses and taverns, again already a source of concern because of the association with loose morals and dubious activities, were to be examined because they were the 'greatest occasion of dispersing the Plague'. Tavern owners were not to admit anyone to their establishment after nine o'clock at night. If successfully implemented then these actions would not only have helped prevent the ravages of the plague but would have controlled the unfavourable activities of the lower ranks.

A particular group of people identified plague victims – the searchers. From at least 1574 local parishes employed searchers as a part of their plague response. The searchers were nearly always women, particularly older women who were already receiving poor relief. Literary historian Richelle Munkhoff has explained that these women would have been among the most conspicuous of local authority figures. As officials working for the parish authorities these women – who usually held a rather lowly position in society – were invested with significant power. Their identification of plague corpses provided the numbers for the Bills of Mortality, the tallies of the dead printed weekly in London from 1593. The bills usually categorised all deaths by putting a total next to each category of illness. Others listed the number of deaths in each parish, noting how many of those died of the plague. The bills had a significant impact on people's daily experiences of the plague. Diarists like Samuel Pepys and Ralph Josselin used them to understand the severity of outbreaks. Josselin recorded throughout 1665 the numbers of dead reported in London and other areas. For example, on August 20 he noted that 'London's visitation said 3880 plague, 5319 all diseases; spread almost over the whole city and much in [the] country; Lord arise & help'. In fact, such was the severity of this outbreak that most contemporary diarists, no matter where they lived in the country, made reference to it in one form or another. Moreover, because the results were listed by parish, as people attempted to shun those with disease the bills provided a geographical map of where to avoid.

Searchers had the power to call for a quarantine if they identified a living plague victim. As the *Orders* outlined: 'these Examiners be sworn by the Alderman, to enquire and learn from time to time what Houses in every Parish be visited, and what persons be sick, and of what Diseases, as near as they can inform themselves.' Intriguingly the use of older women for this role meant that medical practitioners and the authorities must have trusted these women's powers of medical diagnosis. Of course they were in a very dangerous position, one that many others would have avoided, so there was little choice but to trust their diagnosis. The *Orders* suggest that their diagnosis might not always have been accurate. Given the list of symptoms described in *The Plagues Approved Physician* this is unsurprising. To compensate for this the orders suggested that 'upon doubt in that case, to command restraint of access, until it appear what the Disease shall prove'. Whether their diagnosis proved accurate or not, these women were able to quarantine people, thereby threatening livelihoods and lives.

The quarantine is, perhaps, the most well known measure designed to prevent the spread of the pestilence. It was usually called the 'Shutting up' of houses. When a member of a household fell ill with the plague, the house would be sealed with all family members inside, until the infection passed. As the *Orders* explained:

> *AS soon as any man* [or woman] *shall be found by this Examiner, Chirurgion or Searcher to be sick of the Plague, he shall the same night be sequestered in the same house. And in case he be so sequestered, then though he afterwards die not, the House wherein he sickened shall be shut up for a Month, after the use of due Preservatives taken by the rest.*

In 1518 a royal decree said that plague houses in London should be identifiable by a straw bundle hanging at the windows. This was later replaced by the practice of painting a 'Red Cross of a foot long, in the middle of the door' with the words '*Lord have mercy upon us*'. The sight of these locked houses could be quite distressing for residents. During the Great Plague of 1665 Samuel Pepys noted that he was: 'Sad at the news that seven or eight houses in Bazing Hall Street, are shut up of the plague'. While many houses were locked up because a plague victim had been identified within, anyone who entered a property connected with the disease ran the risk of being quarantined themselves. The *Orders* noted that:

> *IF any person shall have visited any man, known to be Infected of the Plague, or entered willingly into any known Infected House, being not allowed: the House wherein he inhabiteth shall be shut up for a certain days by the Examiners direction.*

The practice of shutting up houses was, unsurprisingly, unpopular. Writing in the eighteenth century, Daniel Defoe's fictional account of life during this outbreak claimed that 'all that could conceal their Distempers, did it to prevent their Neighbours shunning and refusing to converse with them; and also to prevent Authority shutting up their Houses.' Defoe's account is meant to be a representation of those times and so it can be taken as a credible account of how it was to live through the plague. Once in force the measure was equally unpopular. Those imprisoned attempted to break out. Defoe recounted one tale of a watchman standing guard at a door while the whole family escaped out of a window on the other side of the building. Family members and friends attempted to circumvent the quarantine, bringing those inside the house food and aid. In theory those inside such houses were supposed to be provided for and constables who were set to watch the houses and ensure the quarantine wasn't broken were able to pass necessary items to those inside. In York in 1550 for example, a weekly rate was introduced to support those in quarantine. Yet, in 1604, the Plague Act gave watchmen the authority to use force to ensure quarantines weren't broken, suggesting that these measures were still controversial. The use of force was perhaps necessary, as things could get violent. Defoe explained that in another instance the local people 'blowed up a Watchman with Gunpowder, and burnt the poor Fellow dreadful', while the poor man lay on the floor injured and crying, the family from the house he was guarding, again, escaped through a window.

Fleeing Physicians

Another controversial response to the plague was that exhibited by physicians themselves. Several historians have noted that one of the core pieces of advice for avoiding the plague was to avoid people and urban centres. Many who could afford it therefore fled the cities and moved to the countryside where the risk of infection was lower. Many of the physicians who catered for this rank of people followed suit, leaving the poorer people of London, and other urban centres, to their fate. This was seen by some as rather selfish and uncharitable.

A side-effect of this movement of physicians out of the capital was that many unlicensed medical practitioners found themselves able to practice plague medicine without as much risk of the Royal College of Physicians criticising or prosecuting them. Once the crisis had passed, several of these empirics and irregular practitioners argued, based on their experience, that they should be more respected. They, after all, had shown courage and charity in helping the poor to brave the ravages of the epidemic. For example, the Society of Apothecaries claimed in the 1630s that they should be allowed to practice medicine because the absence of physicians had compelled them to adopt that role. Individuals made similar arguments. In 1678, the College pursued Mr Russell for being an unlicensed practitioner. He had a lucky escape when the Lord Chamberlain informed them that he had cured people during the great plague. Likewise Thomas Lodge, author of *A Treatise of the Plague* decided to stay and practice during the 1603 outbreak. The son of a Mayor of London, Lodge was very much a Renaissance man, having been a respected lawyer, a prolific author of literature, including poetry, and an adventurer, travelling with Thomas Cavendish to Brazil and other places, before studying for a medical degree in Europe in 1600. This was recognised by Oxford two years later, although his application to join the College of Physicians was denied. Around 1606, Lodge fled to the continent because, as a practising Catholic, he was at risk of prosecution. The chemical physician Thomas O'Dowde also stayed in London, this time in the 1665 outbreak. O'Dowde had apprenticed with an apothecary, so was not a university-trained physician. He claimed to have developed medicines to cure the plague but, according to his daughter Mary Trye in her defence of him published in 1674, he was so preoccupied in treating the sick that he failed to recognise that he too had caught the plague. He died from the disease in August 1665, followed by his wife nine days later. Mary took over from her father and called herself a 'female physician', and ascribed her survival to his medicines.

Fires, Fumes, and Pigeons: Searching for a Cure

Given its ferocity and mortality rate, it is little wonder that people tried a range of remedies to both ward off and cure the disease. The belief that plague was spread by miasma is perhaps the most commonly known amongst modern audiences. Miasmas were bad smells that permeated the body causing disease and ill health. The smell of corruption and decay was thought to cause decay and corruption within the body. One response to plague outbreaks in urban areas was, therefore, to try and clean up the city and remove troublesome smells to other areas. The plague *Orders* republished during one seventeenth-century outbreak argued that 'the sweeping and filth of houses be daily carried away', by specially employed 'Rakers'. The streets were to be kept clean, and each household was to be responsible for the daily cleansing of their own doorstep. In addition, the *Orders* urged that 'no stinking Fish, or unwholesome Flesh, or musty Corn, or other corrupt fruits of what sort soever, be suffered to be sold about the City.'

Maintaining a clean and sweet-smelling home that would ward off the disease was very important. One short medical treatise attributed only to a 'Learned Physician' (although being anonymous this is difficult to qualify), which offered *Present Remedies against the Plague* opened with advice to maintain a healthy fragrant environment. The author recommended that people 'Air your several rooms with Charcoal fires, made in stone pans or Chafing dishes, and not in Chimneys: set your pans in the middle of the Rooms: air every room once a week (at the least) and put into your fire a little quantity of Frankincense, Juniper, dried Rosemary, or of Bay leaves.' This was followed up by the suggestion of a 'Fume of great experience' made from rosemary steeped in strong vinegar.

The body's vulnerability to miasmatic pollutions meant also that people carried sweet-smelling posies and pomanders, which created an aromatic bubble of protection around the body. For example, one recommendation stated that: 'It is very good when one goeth abroad, to have something in their hands to smell too, the better to avoid those noisome stinks, and filthy savors which are in every corner, therefore it is very good to carry in the hand a branch of *Rue, Rosemary, Roses,* or *Camphor.*' Pomanders were portable perfume dispensers. Their name derived from the French *pomme d'amber* (apple of ambergris), as they were originally small balls containing ambergris. Over the era they developed into more elaborate spherical metal containers housing a range of perfumes and could be worn as a necklace or attached to a girdle. Inside there were compartments to hold a range of spices or a sponge dipped in scented water.

Some men and women also took to wearing amulets – or, as they were sometimes called, Plague-cakes – to ward off the disease. These were sometimes made of poisons and hung around the neck to allow the amulet to sit next to the breast and the heart. Francis Herring published a pamphlet in 1604 in which he noted that he had read of some empirics selling amulets made of 'a Toad, Arsenic, or Sublimate'. A toad might seem like an odd choice in this context, but it was explained that its tuberous skin resembled a plague victim covered in lesions. Moreover, toads were thought to eat a lot of worms, which corresponded to the worms sometimes found in the bellies of plague victims. Finally, the toad was thought to be particularly hate-filled, which caused the disease to fear the body of man.

There were several reasons offered for why amulets made of poison might work. W. Kemp's 1665 treatise on surviving the pestilence suggested that: 'Some think that the heart becomes thereby somewhat more familiar and accustomed to poison; and will not so easily be hurt and overcome by it'. Alternatively, the innate heat of poisons like arsenic supposedly dried up noxious humours and so stopped internal putrefaction. Yet again it was said that the amulet drew the poison to itself and intercepted it before it could 'do any mischief to the Heart'. Kemp claimed that this was similar to the commonly stated belief that hot bread and onions would draw all infection in a room into their substance. Not everyone was a believer though; Francis Herring condemned use of these amulets and confidently avowed that: 'I who do not easily believe everything which I read or here, do greatly doubt of the force and nature of those poisons, and do assuredly persuade myself, that they can never produce any such effect'.

In addition to fumigating and wearing amulets, men and women printed, discussed, circulated and recorded in recipe books a whole range of medicines believed to cure the plague. Some of these worked through the humoral model and attempted to rectify the corrupt humours of the body; others worked by transference – drawing the disease out of the body and into another vessel that would subsequently die along with the disease. *The Plague's Approved Physician* claimed that pigeons were particularly efficacious in this regard:

> *Take a Pigeon, and pluck the feathers off her tail, very bare, and set her tail to the sore, and she will draw out the venom till she die; then take another and set too likewise, continuing so till all the venom be*

drawn out, which you shall see by the Pigeons, for they will die with the
venom as long as there is any in it: also chicken or a hen is very good.

The recipe book attributed to Anne Brumwich recommended, amongst others, that walnut water was good for the plague, 'or any infectious diseases'. The water combined 2lbs of walnuts with two handfuls of rue, and 2lbs of figs. Once beaten in a mortar, these ingredients soaked in Sack (a sweet Spanish wine) for an hour, after which some sugar was added. The Brumwich recipe collection, like most, contained numerous different remedies – potentially a means to keep trying to cure someone in the face of little success and therefore a way to mitigate the fear of the disease. On another page of this collection the author revealed their hope that an effective cure existed. The title given for the remedy is 'An Excellent receipt for the plague which did help 600 in York & in one house where 8 were Infected 2 of [them] drank of it & lived the other would not & died'.

The plague was one of the most devastating diseases of this era. It affected people from every background and instilled fear in most. Yet mysteriously the plague began to recede in Europe from about the 1720s. Historians and others have debated why this might have been, but little consensus has been reached. It was once suggested that the replacement of black rats with brown ones reduced the spread of the disease, but this has largely been dispelled. Other explanations have been that quarantine measures were successful, although as we have seen this is debatable. Some suggest that changes to major travel routes interrupted the passage of the disease into Europe from other parts of the world. Alternatively, some have turned to changing climate to explain the departure of the disease – the early modern era has been described as a little ice age, which ended around the same time as the plague began to lose its grip on Europe. Lastly, it has been suggested that the disease mutated into a less virulent form. Whatever the cause, and it is likely that no single cause can explain the decline, people's fear of the disease did not immediately dissipate and the plague lingered in the popular mind-set as a representation of misery and despair.

Chapter 16

Scrofula: The King's Evil

'This healing touch reviv'd / Her drooping state, and promis'd a long-liv'd Felicity'
— Anon, *Anglia Rediviva*

Throughout early modernity there was one disease that maintained a close connection to the royal family, so much so that its popular name was the King's Evil. This disease was scrofula, also known as struma. It was widely believed that the monarch, from the time of Edward the Confessor in the eleventh century, was imbued with special powers to heal this condition. In imitation of Christ who healed by laying his hands on the sick and infirm, the king would stroke or touch those afflicted with the scrofula to cure them. Anointing the monarch's hands during the coronation was a symbol of their divine right to rule, and, in part, was responsible for the monarch's healing powers. Touching for this disease ended with the death of Queen Anne in 1714.

The Sins of the Nation

Richard Boulton's 1715 book on the subject claimed that the disease varied in its manifestations – according to the place of the disease and the constitution of the patient – so that it was impossible to give a definitive definition of the disorder. Yet most authors agreed that melancholic and phlegmatic humours, forming hard swellings or tumours in the neck and adjoining parts, caused the disease. Scrofula is now known to be a swelling of the lymph nodes caused by the tuberculosis bacillus. Beyond the pathology of the condition, medics and moralists blamed the collective sins of the nation for the manifestation of the disease. For the most part the tumours were painless so, according to a 1687 edition of Paul Barbette's treatise, it was significant if they began to hurt becauase it was a sign that they 'threaten[ed] to become cancerous'. The longer the swellings existed the more difficult they were to cure, and once fixed to the nerves in the throat, a person might lose the power of speech. Barbette also cautioned that the cure of the King's Evil would leave behind 'great Scars'.

A Kingly Cure?

As discussed, medieval monarchs, and the early Tudor monarchs, practiced the royal touch for scrofula. However, the transition to Protestantism occurring at the start of this era made the apparently miraculous nature of this cure problematic. Elizabeth I had an uneasy relationship with the practice, and James I on his ascension to the English throne declared that God alone could perform miracles and so he would not offer to cure people by touch. He must have changed his mind, though, because instead of abandoning it altogether he reformed the ritual of the royal touch to meet his own religious ideas. He emphasised, as Elizabeth had, that he was merely a conduit for God's grace; he was not himself endowed with the ability to cure the sick. Indeed, under the Stuart monarchs the royal touch became ever more popular and thousands of people clamoured to be healed by the kings. Historian Stephen Brogan's 2015 study described how both James and Charles I thus had to put into place measures to attempt to restrict the number of supplicants they saw. How successful these measures were is questionable as both Charles II and James II continued to heal large numbers of their subjects. A manuscript held in the Wellcome Library, London, records that from 8 January 1685 to 20 June 1686, James II touched an astonishing 4,893 for the King's Evil.

Given that this power resided with the 'legitimate' monarch, it is little wonder that people used thaumaturgic powers to support claims of royal lineage. A pamphlet produced in 1686 outlined *The Ceremonies used in the Time of King Henry VII for the Healing of them that be Diseased with King's Evil*, suggesting to readers a continuity in these practices across the reigns of the Tudor and Stuart monarchs. Charles II had healed people while in exile in France as a way of asserting his own divine kingship. Moreover, in 1680 stories circulated that the Duke of Monmouth, illegitimate son of Charles II, had cured 20-year-old Elizabeth Parcet, a poor widow's daughter, who had suffered – or as it was said 'languished' – for over ten years with the disease. This was not a ceremonial act; the girl took it upon herself to 'touch' the Duke as he passed her (perhaps a clever twist in the story to emphasise the powers were innate in the Duke and not for show). Henry Clark, author of a pamphlet about the events published at the time, declared that the girl:

> pressed in among a Crowd of People, and caught him by the hand, his
> Glove being on, and she had a Glove likewise to cover her wounds, she not
> being herewith satisfied with this first attempt of touching his Glove only,
> but her mind was, she much touch some part of his bare skin; she waiting

his coming forth, intended a second attempt: the poor Girl, thus betwixt hope and fear waited his motion [...] rent off her Glove that was clung to the Sores in such hast, that broke her Glove, and brought away not only the sores, but the skin: the Duke's Glove, as providence would have it, the upper part hung down, so that his hand-wrist was bare; she pressed one and caught him by the bare hand-wrist with her running hand.

The Duke said to her 'God bless you', and she felt her success. She was convinced that she would recover having done this, but was reproved by her mother for her bold actions. According to the pamphlet, her sores dried up soon after and her vision, impeded by a swelling in her eye, returned. Only a year later, even more spurious claims circulated that the Duke's half-sister, Madam Fanshaw, had healed 'an Apple-woman's Son', 19-year-old Jonathan Trott. According to those who claimed this event had taken place, Jonathan's mother had initially intended to take him to Windsor to be touched by the King. However, the night before their journey she heard a voice in her dream tell her to have Mrs Fanshaw touch her son instead. Not everyone was convinced of the truth of these tales though. The author of a pamphlet deriding these claims as 'lying libel' said that it was silly of the Duke's supporters to advocate such tales in order to bolster a sense of legitimacy in his claims to the throne. It was evident he said, that this power belonged to the Crown not to its heirs, and that coronation would endow a previously ungifted person with such healing powers.

Despite the controversy, it was the case that stories like this weren't always dismissed, suggesting that a proportion of the population were willing to believe that this was not specifically a royal gift. Valentine Greatrakes, the Irish healer who attempted to cure Lady Anne Conway's inveterate headaches had, shortly after the Restoration in 1660, come to the 'strange persuasion' that he was blessed with the ability to cure the King's Evil. Greatrakes initially concealed his gifts, and when he confided in his wife she promptly told him that it was his 'strange imagination'. Yet, it seems, he could not help himself and experimented with his gifts, eventually gaining a reputation as a person who could heal by touch alone. This led him inevitably into trouble. When it came to the attention of the monarchy that he was curing scrofula, the preserve of the king, he was summoned to Dublin to face interrogation by the clerical hierarchy. There he was admonished to stop stroking, but continued to employ his gifts.

He then travelled to England to treat Lady Anne's headaches. Some who encountered him were convinced of his gifts: Henry More, who met Greatrakes while he was at the Conways' home Ragley Hall, claimed that his powers were evidenced by the fact that his 'Body as well as his Hand and

Urine, had a sort of Herbous Aromatic Scent'. His supporters often noted that his body odour was a sign of his inner piety and morality, which helped convince people that God had indeed blessed him with genuine healing powers. Not everyone was convinced though, as Peter Elmer's 2013 book on this colourful character shows; when he was eventually summoned to court to display his gifts, the king was reportedly unimpressed that Greatrakes could not heal the courtier-poet Sir John Denham, who was 'distracted'.

While Valentine Greatrakes might have been the most notorious non-royal 'stroker' of the early modern period, he was not alone. Those whose birth made them unusual were also thought to be endowed with thaumaturgic powers. Medical pamphlet writer John Peachi described how one young man was 'stroked by seven *Seventh* sons'. Elizabeth Parcet had allegedly been taken '10 or 11 Miles' from her home to a 'Seventh Son' before her encounter with the Duke. Seven was a mystical number in early modern thought, leading to the belief that seventh sons, and sometimes seventh daughters, had particular occult qualities. People also used the hands of hanged men to cure a variety of bodily swellings, including scrofula. People waited at the gallows and asked the executioner to stroke the bodies of patients with the deceased hand. The *Gentleman's Magazine* of April 1758 recounted that during the hanging of brothers James and Walter White at Kennington Common, 'a child about nine months old was put into the hands of the executioner, who nine times, with one of the hands of each of the dead bodies, stroked the child over the face' to cure a swelling he had.

Mundane Medical Remedies

Those who could not access the healing touch employed humoral cures for the disease. Ambroise Paré recommended that those prone to scrofulous tumours should live on a 'slender diet'. He reasoned that a lack of nourishment would cause the body to turn on the tumours and consume them. Alternatively, he suggested that an ointment usually used to treat syphilis should be applied to the swellings. If this did not do the trick then other topical applications might help the suppuration – or the forming of pus – and once the humours within the swelling had turned to pus, they would either break forth naturally or a surgeon could make an incision. Paré was a surgeon himself and so also noted that '*scrophulae*' that had 'no deepe roots' could be 'pulled and cut away' surgically, although great care should be taken not to 'violate or hurt with our instrument, the jugular veines, the sleep arteries, or recurrent nerves' of the neck.

Some patients were perhaps wary of the potential for a surgeon to nick a major blood vessel causing a 'great efflux of blood', and so may have stuck to non-invasive prescriptions. Not all of these had to come from a surgeon or physician, who were of course financially out of reach for many. A pamphlet published in 1697 by the apothecary Maurice Tobin, framed as a letter to the surgeon William Cowper, claimed that one Timothy Beaghan was famous for curing the King's Evil. This pamphlet hyperbolically opened with the claim that, 'it was thought nothing but a Supernatural Virtue granted to Kings from Heaven could entirely Cure it', but that it was apparent that Beaghan, who had recently been killed in the Five Bells tavern in the Strand, had cured numerous patients. Beaghan's wonder-cure was a diet drink, pills, and if necessary, surgical intervention. This secret remedy originally belonged to Beaghan's wife who made her living curing scrofulous patients. After her death the impoverished Beaghan used the remedy to earn a living; this was fortunate, since he had lost his leg while a sergeant in the Earl of Litchfield's regiment, making it difficult for him to earn a living any other way. The author of the pamphlet pointed out that this was no mean feat given that he had 'no Experience in the secret, [and] no Skill in Medicines, nor in their Preparations'. He did encounter one snag in his money-making endeavour though. He was so poor and 'despicable' that potential patients would not believe he could cure them. He therefore teamed up with Tobin, who began to recommend patients to him. Indeed Tobin was much surprised 'to see Ulcers and Fistulas healed, most obstinate Tumours dissolved, the Mass of Blood sweetened and rectified, corroded Bones cleansed and made sound, little Scrophulous Children, all Emaciated and at Death's door, miraculously Recovered.'

Tobin played upon that fact that scrofula was difficult to cure, thus emphasising the marvel of his treatments. He was not alone in doing so. As we have already seen, John Peachi was fond of making claims about the efficacy of particular plants in curing particular diseases and he, of course, had one in mind for the King's Evil. The Malabar Nut, he claimed, was 'Beyond anything yet found out' for easing scrofula. Peachi praised this remedy elucidating that:

> *The strange and almost miraculous Cures, that I have known wrought by the* Malabar *Nut, in the King's Evil, would fill a man with wonder and Amazement: And indeed, to see so many Tumours under the Throat, and in other parts, to fall and disappear; to see running Sores dried up, and weak Limbs restored to their Strength, upon the use of such a plain simple Medicine, is exceeding remarkable.*

Peachi explained that these dramatic cures were possible because the nut rectified the blood and altered the offending bodily humours. It mended the liver and the spleen and restored the digestive ferment of the stomach and bowels, thereby modifying the quality of the whole body and making it wholesome. The use of this simple remedy, he claimed, worked in a young lad where the royal touch had failed.

Some remedies were more mundane. William Salmon's 1707 edition of the *Pharmacopoeia Londinensis* recommended a cataplasm (a poultice or a plaster) of kidney beans, the oil of vervain, figwort and barley. While Thomas Fuller's *Pharmacopoeia Extemporanea* (1730) suggested that water of millipedes – made by taking a pint and a half of live millipedes, orange and lemon peel, white bread and nutmeg distilled in juice of scabious and cleavers, and whey – was a useful remedy. This, like Peachi's nuts, was intended to change the blood. It was also designed to promote urination and clear the nerves. Fuller also recommended burdock water, which could also contain forty or fifty millipedes 'mashed, washed and squeezed out.'

Remission and Recovery

Throughout the era the potential to recover from scrofula was a little ambiguous. Yet, medics now and in the early modern period were aware that scrofula could go into remission. J.A. Browne noted in his treatise on the disease that some criticised the royal touch for failing to permanently cure the condition. He thereby demonstrated an acknowledgement that the disease could fade and return of its own accord. Likewise another medical writer noted that 'Nature' who was the 'Lady physician of all Diseases' sometimes caused the disease to spontaneously disappear, allowing for a form of remission, if not recovery.

Medical writers simultaneously noted that the disease was easy to cure if attended to quickly, by amending the diet and redressing the humours, but difficult to cure if neglected for any length of time. Many of the cases that came before the monarchy were precisely those that were longstanding, and not always through neglect. Many patients had already sought treatment, which had failed, when they turned to the king, or queen, for help. So while the disease appeared pernicious and persistent, medical authors wrote that ultimately it could be cured, if by nothing else then by God acting through the person of the monarch.

Chapter 17

Scurvy: Scabs, Spots, and Stinking Breath

'This is but a scurvy Tune for your Hymenical Song, Sir'
                                                    – Aphra Behn

Thy scurvy scornful rolling Eyes
Of my heart ne're shall make a prize,
Thy beetle Brows and tallow face
Makes young men run from thee a pace;
Thy hair is like my Sorrel's mane
The words I speak are very plain,

So went the fourth stanza of the seventeenth-century ballad *The Young Lover, or, a New Way of Wooing*, in which an 'honest lad' rebuked a 'proud lass' who took pleasure in mocking the young men of Northamptonshire. His opening salvo was to mention the maids 'scurvy scornful rolling Eyes'. Used as an insult, people regularly conflated scurvy and 'scurfy', in part because one of the symptoms of scurvy was spots. In this way these terms were designed to bring to mind the scabby nature of diseased skin and a sense of a person being sorry, worthless, and contemptible. Samuel Pepys used the term in his diary to designate things that were less than savoury. On 8 March 1661 he mentioned that while having a 'cup of ale at the Swan' with Sergeant Pierce, the man had told him 'many more scurvy stories of him and his brother Ralph, which troubles me to hear of persons of honour as they are.'

Throughout the era numerous medical texts were produced that specifically discussed and described scurvy. Everard Maynwaring, a physician originally from Gravesend who was created MD of the University of Dublin in 1655, produced one such text, *Morbus Polyrhizos et Polymorphæus, a Treatise of the Scurvy* (1665). Maynwaring established himself as a physician and practitioner in London and in 1665 was put in charge of the pest-house (plague hospital) for the poor in Middlesex. In terms of medical philosophy, he followed the chemico-medical ideas of Jean Baptiste van Helmont. Most people think of scurvy as a disease of sailors, and indeed in the early modernity it was as well, but it was (hopefully, unlike today) a condition widely experienced by those living on land as well as those at sea. This, in part, was because it was often confused with other diseases, notably syphilis. Maynwaring's treatise opened with the observation that '*Amongst the complaints of the diseased none more frequently mentioned than the Scurvy*'. In describing the disease Maynwaring was clear that the name 'scurvy' could be applied to a range of diseases that manifested as pocks or spots on the skin, including venereal disease. He also said that it could be applied to dropsy, epilepsy, convulsions, and pleurisy. However, as a disease in its own right, he used the name the '*Scorbute*', or in Latin, '*Scorbutus*'.

A short pamphlet produced some thirty years after Maynwaring's text by a M. Bromfield – designed to sell 'Bromfield's Pills' – claimed that scurvy 'chiefly proceed[ed] from Melancholy bred by distempers of the Stomach or Spleen'. These crude melancholic humours were sluggish and so stayed in the arteries and veins causing a 'grievous Fermentation', which produced vapours that assaulted the brain and the heart. All together this created a malignant putrefaction of the body's melancholy causing a range of symptoms:

> *Giddiness in the head, sudden flushings, heat and redness in the face and body, putrefaction and stinking of the mouth and gums, Toothache, stinking breath, blackness and looseness of the teeth, want of digestion, much wind, and unsavoury belchings [...] obstructions of respiration, or shortness of Breath, and straightness of the Breast, &c. The body is dull and heavy, and in the legs are spots, sometimes red, purple, black, or blue: There are also violent pains in the head, shoulders, arms, fingers, belly, thighs, knees, legs, ankles, feet and toes.*

Bromfield, like Maynwaring, lamented that the numerous and varied symptoms meant that scurvy was often misdiagnosed – in this case he claimed it was often mistaken for gout, but he noted that in some cases it was also diagnosed as dropsy or consumption. Of course Bromfield's pills were themselves supposed to treat scurvy, dropsy, agues, and a range of other ills so, rather conveniently, they would be applicable even if the patient had been misdiagnosed.

The Mariners' Malady

As noted above, the connection between scurvy and those who worked at sea is longstanding. The Greeks and Romans acknowledged this connection and one of the names for the disease was *Purpura nautica*. Throughout the age of discovery, the world was expanding and sea voyages were becoming ever longer. Extended time at sea and the concurrent reliance on long-lasting victuals meant that scurvy became a much more common condition in the early modern period. Texts produced by sea surgeons and medical practitioners that dealt specifically with the ailments of sailors regularly noted that it was one of the more common diseases they faced, along with the flux. The second printing of William Cockburn's *Sea Diseases* (1736), for example, claimed that 'we find the *Scurvy, Fevers*, and *Fluxes*, a *Diarrhoea* particularly, and a *Dysentry*, the most genuine Diseases at Sea.' The surgeon John Moyle noted in his medical book, *An Abstract of Sea-Chirurgery* (1686), that he had experienced the disease when travelling to Newfoundland. By the time Bromfield was trying to sell his patent pills it was clearly well known that sailors were liable to the disease. He wrote that his pills were 'a precious Medicine for Mariners, and such as use the Seas, to whom the Scurvy, and many other Diseases are very incident; partly from bad Airs, Sea Fogs, Sudden Heats and Colds, much Salt Diet; and sometimes from excessive drinking of Foreign and unfrequented Liquors.'

As hinted at here, although Bromfield, and others, listed diet as a cause of the disease, the British Navy believed that the disease was the result of damp sea air and the miasma, or foul air, found below decks. Moreover, some held that lazy and sluggish sailors were the more likely to develop the condition. William Cockburn was of this persuasion opining that: 'Lazy Temper among some Seamen, and most of the pressed Land-men [those men forced into service by a press gang], is the true Original of the genuine Scurvies that are commonly to be met with at Sea.'

Some authors were more insistent that diet, and in particular citrus fruits, was the crucial factor in understanding the development and cure of the disease. Sir Hugh Plat's 1607 instructions *Certain Philosophical Preparations of Food and Beverage for Seamen*, listed food for sailors and commended lemon juice to preserve against scurvy. William Cockburn likewise explained that:

> *The* Scurvy *being generated by the Salt Provisions, altogether unavoidable at Sea, makes one of the constant Diseases in Navies, and is the Reason why it seldom appears in Camps. On the contrary, the putting the Seamen ashore off of the mentioned Diet, proves their absolute Cure. This was very conspicuous in 1695, when we were to be one Month in Torbay.*

At this time, Cockburn claimed, he fought to have tents erected on shore where the sick were treated. He moved 100 'perfect moving Skeletons' into these tents where they had fresh provisions including carrots, turnips and other '*green Trade*'. These men recovered in time to put to sea. In many of these texts we see healers recommending lemon and orange juice. John Moyle's book explained that the cure should be based on 'diet and drink' that included 'fresh Vegetables', green fruit, 'Lemons, Apples, or Roots and Herbs, as Salad.' Despite the pronouncements of those like Cockburn, Moyle and Robert Boyle (who also publically declared that lemons cured the disease), traditional medical thinking did not readily adopt the idea. One historian has posited that this was because in humoral theory, diseases were caused by the *presence* of something (usually corrupt or vitiated) and so many could not get their heads around the idea of a disease caused by the *absence* of something.

James Lind and Clinical Trials

Just after the period we are interested in, James Lind was credited with improving understandings of the disease. In 1747, in what has sometimes been called the first controlled clinical medical study, Lind took twelve patients with the disease and tested the effects of different diets on their condition. All the patients resided on the same ship, the *Salisbury*, and were all fed water-gruel sweetened with sugar in the morning, mutton broth, pudding or boiled biscuits with sugar for lunch, and barley and raisin, rice and currants, or sago and wine for supper. They were given cider each day to drink and took twenty-five drops of *elixir vitriol* (sulphuric acid) three times a day. The patients were split into several pairs and each pair was given an additional element to their diet. Two men were given two spoonfuls of vinegar three times a day. Two of the sickest patients were ordered to drink half a pint of seawater every day. Two others each had two oranges and one lemon a day. The final two patients partook of an electuary advocated by a hospital surgeon three times a day. It was made with garlic, mustard seed, balsam of Peru, and gum myrrh; to drink they had barley water with tamarind and cream of tartar. As we would expect, the two patients consuming the citrus fruits recovered quickly and visibly – one was reported as being ready for duty after just six days. Lind concluded that the oranges, and then the cider he had prescribed had the best effects. Yet in the face of all of this evidence, the British Admiralty didn't issue the order for all men-of-war to have a supply of lemon juice until 1795.

Cochlearia Curiosa

At the same time naval and medical men were discussing and experimenting with the virtues of lemon juice, medics, including some of a more spurious nature, were offering remedies based on the plant *cochlearia*. Leipzig physician Valentin Andreas Moellenbrock's book on the plant was translated into English in 1676. It explained the naming origins and use of the plant. The name, he explained, derived from the fact that 'its leaves are turned up, and hollowed round, nearly expressing the outward shape of a Spoon.' Its vernacular name, based on its use, was 'scurvygrass'. There was evidently some disagreement amongst botanists as to whether it was the same plant as bistort, but Moellenbrock strongly refuted this. Part of the confusion might have been because there were different kinds of scurvygrass. Robert Turner's 1664 herbal claimed that there was sea scurvygrass (also known as Dutch scurvygrass) and garden scurvygrass. In its qualities, the plant was described as being hot and dry, like cress. It was predominantly used to treat scurvy but was also thought to be beneficial for agues, evacuating cold, clammy, and phlegmatic humours from the liver, blood, and spleen, and for reducing swellings, while the juice of the plant also eased ulcers and sores in the mouth, cleared spots and helped scars.

By the 1680s several sellers were advertising 'Spirits' of scurvygrass through handbill notices. Both Robert Bateman and George Blagrave offered a 'plain' and a 'golden' spirit. Bateman claimed that the spirits were different because the first purged the body by urine, the second by stool. Blagrave's advert revealed at least eighteen different people in London sold the spirits, including booksellers, grocers, printers, a milliner, a perfumer, and two cheesemongers. At the same time another pamphlet offered a remedy that 'far exceeds the common distilled Spirit of *Scurvy-Grass*' in curing the scurvy and its associated diseases. This 'Elixir *of* Scurvy-grass' incorporated horseradish and both sea and garden scurvygrass with an appropriate liquid according to the '*Spagerick* [chemical] *Art*'. It could be purchased for one shilling a glass from Mr Joseph Sabbarton at the Norwich Coffeehouse or, again, from a range of sellers and merchants around the city.

Domestic Cures

Some collectors of medical recipes also relied upon scurvygrass in their cures. The book of Sir Thomas Osborne included several remedies for the scurvy, one of which, 'A water to cleanse the Blood and cure the Scurvy' used 'both of garden and Sea Scurvy grass'. But a book belonging to Mary Chantrell and several others, dated to 1690, took a different approach. The book includes a recipe titled 'A powder to keep your Gums and teeth free from scurvy and to Preserve them sound in your head'. This remedy included the ever popular and versatile – if the remedies recited in this book are to be believed – earthworms. As with other remedies, the author specified that these should be 'fresh out of the Garden'. Once cleansed and slowly dried over, or near to, the fire, the producer of the remedy needed to beat them and sieve the resultant powder. The final product could be kept 'in a little Box or Galley pot near [the] fire' and rubbed onto the teeth and gums when necessary. Elizabeth Godfrey's book also included a rub for the gums made from a range of herbs and plants, suggesting that the effects of the disease on the mouth were a particular source of concern.

Although it was James Lind's experiments in the eighteenth century that really changed the way in which scurvy was treated, particularly by the navy, these various remedies show that experience and observation had already proved that diet, citrus fruit, and plants like scurvygrass, were the key to curing the condition. They may not have been able to square this with their notions of health and disease, but in an era where empirical evidence was becoming more and more crucial to medical practice, this didn't stop them.

Chapter 18

Smallpox: Red Pustules and Scarlet Cloth

'How full of the smallpox she is, what ails she to stamp thus?'
– Thomas Dekker

The disease of smallpox, prevalent in early modernity, was finally eradicated in the twentieth century. An incredibly common disease, it attacked royalty and the poorest indiscriminately. On 10 October 1562, when she was in her late twenties, Elizabeth I contracted the disease and became seriously ill, causing a constitutional crisis in the process. While Elizabeth made a full recovery, apart from some scarring, her waiting woman, Lady Mary Sidney, who caught the disease from her, was so disfigured she retired from court. Elizabeth's great rival Mary, Queen of Scots, also had this disease in her childhood, but much less severely than her cousin. In the early 1600s, the notorious Lady Katherine Howard, countess of Suffolk, also retired from public life after losing her looks following a bout of smallpox. She relied on her beauty to advance her fortunes, had long been rumoured to be a lover of Sir Robert Cecil, and was in the pay of the Spanish as a spy. In 1619 she was tried by the Star Chamber on counts of bribe-taking and even spent ten days in the Tower of London. It was later that same year that she came down with smallpox, which ruined the beauty she relied on and ended her time in the public eye. Royalty were still contracting the disease at the end of the seventeenth century when Lady Anne Stuart, later Queen Anne survived the disease at the age of 12 in 1677; her infant step-brother Charles was not so fortunate and died of the disease in December that year.

While the women discussed above survived smallpox, they mostly bore long-term effects and were never the same again. Even so, they were the lucky ones as death rates from this disease were high. On 7 March 1685, the now elderly diarist John Evelyn rushed to his 19-year-old daughter Mary's side after receiving word that she was ill with smallpox. By the next day her physician Dr Short, 'the most approved & famous Physician of all his Majesty's Doctors', warned Evelyn that his daughter needed greater help than was available. The disease, he said, had moved to her lungs and in his opinion, 'she could not escape'. Mary received the sacrament and, as Evelyn wrote, 'bore the remainder of her sickness with extraordinary patience, and piety & with more than ordinary resignation.' She passed away on 14 March to his 'unspeakable sorrow & Affliction'. Similarly, the next year, William and Isabel Scaife published an account of their daughters' deaths from smallpox as part of their expression of their Quaker faith. Mary and Barbara fell ill on 30 January that year, having succumbed to smallpox in 'one and the same hour' as one another. As this account shows, even in their earliest days, Quakers were known for their record-keeping. In total, Mary suffered from this disease for six weeks and three days, dying on 13 March 1686, or 'the 13th of the 3rd Month' as her parents' expressed it, in accordance with the Quaker practice of not using traditional names for months. The account describes how Mary, the elder sister, survived Barbara by two weeks, but that she had a fever as a symptom of the disease, which her parents said 'made her extremity the greater'. As survival from smallpox was low, Mary knew she was unlikely to recover and, according to her parents' account, she stressed how willingly she would return to God but she wanted to be sure that if she had done anything to 'offend him' that he would make this 'manifest' before she grew any weaker. Some of her final words were to her mother and recommended that the family should 'go to live near some good Meeting and bring up my Brother amongst Friends', thereby reinforcing her commitment to the Quaker faith.

The antiquary John Aubrey reported in his *Miscellanies upon the Following Subjects* (1696) that 'The Small-Pox is usually in all great Towns: But it is observed at Taunton in Somersetshire, and at Sherburne in Dorsetshire, that at one of them at every Seventh Year, and at the other at every Ninth Year comes a Small-Pox, which the Physicians cannot master.' This means that Aubrey considered that smallpox, like the plague, broke out cyclically. When the disease arrived in an area the effects could be devastating. James Clegg, a dissenting minister from Derbyshire, who also worked as the local physician, noted in his journal in September 1721 that smallpox had broken out in Kinder, and that the first to die from it were the two sons of Francis Gee. Soon some thirty others, including John Froggat's eldest son, 'a youth of high hopes', had died in the outbreak. Clegg noted that most of the families in the area were 'broken' by the outbreak. He was more fortunate when, in November 1721, his family was infected with the disease, which had 'been so fatal to many others'. Six of his children were ill at the same time, but remarkably they all survived; Clegg was a spiritual man who ascribed this to the power of prayer.

Boiling Blood: the Causes of Smallpox

While the early modern period had no understanding of viruses or bacterial infection, that the smallpox was most likely in densely populated areas was well known. One of the earliest treatises in English on the causes of this disease is by Simon Kellwaye and appeared in 1593. Kellwaye's book and ideas were reprinted throughout the seventeenth century under several different names and titles. Kellwaye also saw a likeness with the plague, in that sufferers of one were often susceptible to the other. He began his explanation by confirming the prevalence of this illness: 'I need not greatly to stand upon the description of this disease, because it is a thing well known unto most people, proceeding of adjusted blood mixed with phlegm'. Kellwaye used the prolific medieval medical author and translator known as Avicenna as his authority in his explanations. Avicenna's five volume *Canon of Medicine*, completed around 1025, was a standard text in English medical training, based as it was on the teachings of Galen. Kellwaye described the presentation of the disease:

> as *Avicen* [sic] *witnesseth, which according to both ancient and later writers doth always begin with a fever, then shortly after there arise small red pustules upon the skin throughout all the body, which do not suddenly come forth, but by intermission in some more or less, according to the state and quality of the body infected therewith for in some there arise many little pustules with elevation of the skin, which in one day do increase and grow bigger, and after have a thick matter growing in them.* [The pustules] *do most commonly appear the fourth day, or before the eight day.*

The primary cause of the disease for Kellwaye was corrupt air, or miasma. He explained that 'by alteration of the air in drawing some putrefied and corrupt quality unto it, which doth cause an ebullition [boiling] of our blood'. He used the sixteenth-century Latin works of French physician Jean François Fernel as his source here. In divergence from Fernel, Kellwaye also explained that another theory about the origins of smallpox was that it was reaction to menstrual blood, which was assumed to nourish the infant in the womb. Kellwaye described how this blood mixing with an embryo's own blood could cause this to become overheated too:

> *The efficient cause, is nature or natural heat, which by that menstrual matter mixing itself with the rest of our blood, doth cause a continual vexing and disquieting thereof, whereby an unnatural heat is increased*

in all the body, causing an ebullition of blood, by the which this filthy
menstrual matter is separated from our natural blood, & the nature
being offended and overwhelmed therewith, doth thrust it to the outward
pores of the skin as the excrements of blood: which matter if it be hot and
slimy, then it produceth the pocks, but if dry & subtle, then the measles
or males.

The notion that menstrual blood could cause smallpox in children was accepted into the seventeenth century and midwife Jane Sharp referred to it as a matter of fact in her 1671 text, writing: 'They have epidemical Fevers sometimes that cast forth the Measles, or small Pox; the mother's menstrual blood is the original cause, but the corrupt air stirs it up.'

The idea that some force, either corrupt air or indeed menstrual blood imbibed *in utero,* caused the blood to boil and erupt in this skin disease was the reason Kellwaye also thought a propensity to the disease was hereditary: 'because few or none do escape it, but that either in their youth, ripe age, or old age, they are infected therewith.' He then went on to draw on another sixteenth-century medic, Italian physician Girolamo Fracastoro, considered an expert in epidemic diseases, who 'witnesseth this disease is very contagious and infectious, as experience teacheth us.' The two reasons it was thought to be so infectious are firstly the effects of external matter on the blood, and secondly a hereditary predisposition that caused it to run through some families, as they were linked with the same blood. In 1666 Thomas Sydenham, a man sometimes called the English Hippocrates, published a book on fevers in Latin which was considered a seminal work on the topic. Indeed, this book was posthumously translated into several English versions in the 1690s. Although Sydenham used Fracastoro's thesis, and outlined clearly the duration of the illness and how pockmarks came out between days four to seven, as Kellwaye had explained, he also stated that the disease lasted from the first signs of illness to recovery for some thirty-one to forty-one days, depending on the individual.

Side Effects

Medical writers knew that the eyes were prone to damage by smallpox. Simon Kellwaye advised the use of a mixture of rosewater and breast milk mixed with a little myrrh as eyewash; he also recommended cold cloths soaked in rosewater applied to the eyes to draw out the pustules and sooth the skin around the eyes. John Hall took steps to protect the eyes of one young patient, Thomas Holyoak, with a *collyrium* or eye-salve made from the herb eye-bright and rose water administered by a feather frequently throughout the day.

Diseases like smallpox were also thought to make a woman liable to miscarry and in her trial for infanticide on 27 February 1684 Elizabeth Stafford used this as part of her defence. Elizabeth was accused of having delivered a baby boy on 19 February and of throwing the infant into the 'house of easement', or toilet, where it suffocated under the waste (excrement, urine and 'other filth'). Instead, Elizabeth and her witnesses argued, she was only about five months pregnant, suffering from smallpox and 'did by that illness Miscarry'. In a similar case Jane Langworth was accused of infanticide, and claimed to be suffering from smallpox when she delivered her baby alone. Jane gave birth to a girl on 13 December 1684, but admitted that she strangled the child with her apron string to stop it crying, and then hid its body in a trunk. Her defence was 'ignorance', presumably that she was so unwell she didn't know what she was doing. The fact that Elizabeth Stafford produced a husband to show that the child was lawfully conceived had more influence on the court at the Old Bailey than the other factors, and she was duly acquitted. Jane also insisted that she was married, but couldn't produce a husband at the trial. She was convicted under 'the Statute of King James' which ordered 'death to any that shall be delivered of an unlawful Issue dead and conceal it', or the 1624 statute, which presumed the guilt of single women who concealed a birth. Jane was duly found guilty of murder and sentenced to death.

'Suffer Him Not to Sleep': Treating Smallpox

A curious aspect of the treatment of smallpox was that patients were often wrapped in red cloth. When Elizabeth I contracted smallpox in 1562 her physicians placed a red cloth over the windows. This was supposed to act as a barrier to harsh light to help prevent scaring. She was also enveloped in a red cloth. In addition to sleeping in a bed hung with red curtains, or hanging red curtains in the windows, patients were supposed to wear red clothing. The English translation of Felix Platter's medical text book, published in 1664, claimed of this method that: 'The vulgar think, the beholding red things, makes the Pustules red, and therefore cover them with scarlet.' Given that the appearance of pustules signified the breaking of the fever and evacuation of toxins from the body, wearing red was designed to hasten the disease's progress towards cure.

Simon Kellwaye considered that there were two main ways to treat this disease: first, bloodletting to help the body expel the overheated blood that would otherwise go on to erupt in the pustules, and second, treatments to protect the body from further harm. If bloodletting was contraindicated (such as was the case for the very young, when it was thought to do more harm than good), then a clyster or enema was recommended. To make this, Kellwaye advised the reader to reduce three pints of water with barley and violet leaves until it was half the volume. Cooled until it was just warm, the liquid was injected into the rectum. After it was expelled the sufferer was gently rubbed with warm cloths to encourage the skin to remove further waste. He stressed that the carer must 'always keep the sick warm and suffer him not to sleep, or permit very little until the pocks or measles do appear.'

John Hall and other physicians employed different cures. Hall treated Thomas Farnham of Leicester for smallpox by giving him a draft of opium and hartshorn, both of which have sedative effects. He also treated 10-year-old Thomas Holyoak in 1626 with opiates and fennel water, primarily to relieve the back pain and stomach ache that Thomas suffered as part of the illness. He also gave him a milk and plantain-water gargle to ease his sore throat, with pomegranate syrup, which Hall considered to be an excellent remedy for strengthening the 'lungs, throat, mouth and breast'. He also stressed that the patient was to be confined to bed with a fire in his chamber. Thomas survived and went on to be a doctor when he grew up. A hundred years later, James Clegg was carrying out similar procedures. His journal entry from 10 September 1725, relates how family friend Elizabeth Bagshaw asked him to make the long journey from Oaks to London to attend her second son Adam, who was dangerously ill. The journey involved three overnight stops, and when he arrived Adam was 'very full of smallpox of a bad kind'. Famous physician Richard Mead was sent for and applied blisters to the skin in order to draw out the disease, against Clegg's views. The boy was given cordials, but Clegg was again overruled in the use of sleeping potions, which he wanted to give. He did prevail in giving a clyster, since Adam had not passed any stools for a fortnight but this was not successful. Adam became delirious and died on 19 September; Clegg accompanied the body home and arrived back a week later.

Offended Skin: Reducing the Scarring

Even with all the privileges of rank, there was no escaping the fact that smallpox could leave a survivor with very bad scarring. Indeed, Elizabeth I wore thick makeup and a wig, it is said, because of the damage the virus caused to her skin and scalp when she recovered from it in her thirtieth year. In the eighteenth century, Lady Mary Wortley Monatgu lost her eyelashes permanently after contracting the disease in her mid-twenties. Naturally there was interest in any treatments people could try to reduce this scarring. John Hall advised patients to anoint their faces with salad oil (olive oil) to stop the risk of scarring. Hannah Woolley's household compendium, *The Accomplish'd Lady's Delight* (1675), includes a whole subsection of 'beautifying waters', which she claimed would 'take away spots in the face after smallpox'. She started with a simple lemon and bay salt (sea salt) wash, which would have a natural exfoliation effect on the skin, before moving on to an ointment. This was manufactured by grinding oil of almonds or lilies in a mortar with some capon grease and goat fat with a scruple of bryony (a plant related to the cucumber) and *ireos* (iris) roots. To this was added some scented water a little at a time to produce the right consistency for dabbing on the spots. William Salmon's *Family Dictionary* (1695) offered a more pragmatic treatment of bacon dripping beaten in water for fifteen minutes until all the offensive smell was gone, and then scented with rosewater. Kept in a gallipot or small jar, this could be applied when the sores were still raw in order to prevent scarring.

Another side effect of this disease was pitting in the skin and Woolley described how an alternating regime of a vinegar wash one day, and a bran and mallow wash the next for around twenty days to a month could help smooth these out. For any residual redness, she advised a facemask-type jelly preparation formed from barley, beans, and lupines, boiled and reduced down, and applied several times a day for three or four days. Her final suggestion for smallpox-related redness involved making a distillation from various herbs, lemon pulp, and chopped up calf's foot in a glass still. Survivors of smallpox who lived near Hatton Garden, London, could save themselves the trouble of making up a beauty treatment by visiting someone described as a gentlewoman who lived at the Blue Ball in Little Kerby Street. Here they could buy an 'incomparable wash for the face', which would not only remove wrinkles and freckles but was especially good for people recently 'prejudiced by the smallpox'.

The Beginning of the End for Smallpox

A method of inoculation emerged in Europe from the late seventeenth century; the procedure now known as variolation, but known then as 'ingrafting', involved taking the infectious matter from a sufferer, and using a piece of thread applying it to a small cut on the skin, bandaging it over until it healed. Reports of this treatment reached England in the early eighteenth century and an account of the concept was given to the Royal Society in 1714. One of earliest proponents of this system was the English aristocrat, Lady Mary Wortley Montagu. Her brother died of smallpox in 1713 and, as mentioned above, she too suffered from it two years later when she was in her mid-twenties. Her personal experience of the disease, perhaps, gave her added impetus in her pioneering efforts to encourage people to take up this preventative method. Lady Mary lived in Constantinople, modern-day Istanbul, while her husband worked as the British ambassador. She wrote to describe how smallpox had been rendered harmless on the continent because large numbers of people went through ingrafting, in a letter to her friend Sarah Chiswell, who would herself die of the same disease in 1726. In Constantinople she saw the success of the method performed annually by two elderly, Greek, itinerant healing women, and she resolved to have her young son inoculated. The surgeon Charles Maitland performed the surgery in 1718, and went on to promote the method himself. Because of her status, the newspapers picked up the story and it was the subject of much discussion in England that year. Once Princess Caroline had reassured herself of the safety of the treatment, such that she felt safe to have her own children inoculated, the procedure effectively had the royal seal of approval and became more mainstream. It still remained controversial and was not universally supported, but Lady Mary remained a lifelong advocate. Eventually Edward Jenner, who himself received variolation as a young child in the mid-eighteenth century, would develop an inoculation method based on cowpox sores, which paved the way to the eventual eradication of the disease in the twentieth century.

Part Four

REPRODUCTIVE MALADIES

Chapter 19

Greensickness: The Virgin's Disease

'Out you green sickness baggage, out you tallow face'
– William Shakespeare

As much of the medical treatment in this book shows, keeping the body in a balanced state was considered to be key to good health. When children were growing it was thought that they used up all their blood in growth, which is why it was extremely unusual to see bloodletting recommended for prepubescents. Once fully grown, medical theory argued that girls amassed blood in their bodies that they did not burn off through activity, causing them to have menstrual periods: a form of natural purge. Girls were expected to have their first period at around the age of 14, give or take a couple of years. Jane Sharp explained the usual assumption in 1671 that menstrual periods 'begin commonly at fourteen years old'. John Freind, author of the first book dedicated solely to menstruation called *Emmenologia,* published in Latin in 1703 and translated into English by Thomas Dale in 1729, expanded on these ideas. Freind wrote that: 'The menstrous Purgation, or a flux of Blood issuing from the Uterus every Month, usually begins its Periods at the *Second Septenary*, and terminates at the *Seventh*, or the Square of the number seven'. So put simply, Freind expected periods to start at the age of 14 and to end at 49, when the natural drying processes of ageing would render them unnecessary.

If a young woman didn't begin to menstruate at the expected time people became concerned because, as Jane Sharp explained, 'if the blood be stopt, in that it cannot break forth, it will corrupt'. This meant young women were at risk of contracting a disease known as 'the white Fever, the Virgins' Disease, the Pale colour of Virgins, the white Jaundice, but vulgarly the Greensickness', according to *The Practice of Physick* (1655). Greensickness was indeed the colloquial name for this illness and was widely used in society, including by Juliet Capulet's father as an insult, in William Shakespeare's *Romeo and Juliet* (1597 edition), as used in the epigram to this chapter. From the mid-seventeenth century, physicians increasingly used the Latin borrowing of *chlorosis*.

Signs and Symptoms

Lazare Rivière's text considered the long-term prognosis for sufferers to be good, even when the disease went on for a long time. It was, however, one that presented with a myriad of indications, the first of which was appearance: 'The Face and all the Body is pale and white, sometimes of a Lead colour, blue, or green' caused by too much phlegm. If 'Choler or Melancholy be mixed with that phlegm, the colour will be yellowish, greenish or blue'. The second sign was oedema or 'Swelling in the Face and Eye-lids, especially after sleep, because the motive heat [heat caused by motion] being closed and contracted at night'. Legs, feet, and ankles might also swell 'by reason of the abundance of phlegm'. Patients would feel lethargic and sleep a lot, due, Rivière suggested to the humours having fallen to their legs. They might also experience breathing difficulties caused by the thickened, corrupted blood, and so have palpitations and a raised pulse. The patient might also experience headaches 'sometimes in the hinder part of the Head, when the Womb suffers'. In addition, patients went off their food, experiencing 'a great loathing of wholesome meat, by reason of the great collection of Crudities in the Stomach and parts adjacent; and these Humours when they grow worse, cause the Pica, or longing for things that are not to be eaten.' Finally: 'When the evil increaseth, and the Obstructions are multiplied, the Terms [periods] stop, which shows the Disease to be at the height, and confirmed.' Missing periods was the emphatic symptom that separated the disease from the many others that had all the other symptoms.

The anonymous eighteenth-century text *A Rational Account of the Natural Weaknesses of Women* (1716) described a letter the author had apparently received from the father of a young woman experiencing most of the symptoms Rivière had previously described:

> *I shall conclude this Chapter with a letter I received while writing it, from a Gentleman in Hartford, whose Daughter, a young Gentlewoman, about seventeen Years of Age, had never had the Benefit of Nature* [started her periods], *but was almost ruined by the Green-Sickness, being exceeding pale, short breathed, and hardly able to move about, without any Appetite to Food, but desirous of eating Chalk, Cinders, Wall, &c. which she could scarcely be kept from; her affectionate Parents had taken the Advice of several Physicians, and the young Lady took a great many Medicines to no purpose.*

Happily, this physician's own medicine 'Purging Pills and Opening Powder', provided a cure, and the publication includes details of where these could be obtained in case other readers wanted to purchase them.

Purges, Bloodletting, and Intimacy

The primary cause of this disease was blockages in the veins of the uterus, which hindered the flow of blood. As Rivière's *Practice of Physick* explained, the 'Causes of the Obstructions in the Veins of the Womb, and the Hypochondria, are thick, slimy, and crude Humours, coming commonly from evil diet.' As the Introduction described, food was one of the non-natural factors in maintaining health and therefore a bad diet was thought to contribute to the likelihood of contracting certain diseases. As mentioned above, Rivière thought that young women with greensickness experienced *pica*-like cravings like pregnant women experience and so 'these Virgins drink great draughts of Water at bed-time, or in the morning fasting [on an empty stomach]; or eat Vinegar, Herbs, unripe Fruits, Snow, or Ice', thus cooling their bodies too much and causing slime to build up in their veins. Steps to remove the blockage and restore the humoral balance were needed. When Northamptonshire gentlewoman Elizabeth Isham wrote her memoirs around 1640, as a spiritual reflection, she noted how when she was in her early teens in the 1620s 'I still looked ill some thinking I had the green sickness.' To try and cure her, her father made her run up and down house stairs, normally referred to as 'pairs of stairs' in this period, 'twelve times & and to rest me once'. According to *The Practice of Physick* people who 'sleep too much, or are very idle, as Seamstresses, which by sitting still all day are very cold' were liable to greensickness. Exercise was thought to excite the blood and so combatted coolness brought on by idleness. By the time Elizabeth was 16 she noted, she was 'growing out of the green sickness [and so] was not so dull as before.'

Rivière explained that the first treatment was some gentle purges to try and cleanse the liver. Somerset apothecary and surgeon John Westover accordingly noted how, on 16 March 1697, 'Robert Porch of Wedmore [became a] debtor for medicine for his daughter being lame and for want of her courses [periods]. [I] sent for her one dose of jalap to purge and ordered her to come to be blooded at the coming of the moon', in accordance with the belief that young women menstruated at the new moon. As this case note suggests, if purges didn't work, then bloodletting was next: 'Then open a Vein, if the Disease be not very old, and the Maid very much without blood, and inclining to an evil habit. Let the Vein of the Arm be opened first, although the Terms [periods] be stopped; for if then you draw blood from the Foot'. In cases of absent periods letting blood from the ankles had been recommended since ancient times, with the idea being that this would encourage blood to flow past the womb, giving the uterine veins a kick-start. If this didn't work, then Rivière recommended a warm herbal bath:

> Take of *Marshmallow Roots, Lilly Roots, Elecampane, Bryony, wild Cucumber, of each two pound: Mallows, Violets, Mercury, Pennyroyal, Feverfew, Balm, of each four handfuls: Linseed and Fenugreek beaten, of two ounces: boil them in spring Water for a Bath. Let her go into it warm twice in a day, not sweating, long before and after meat, for two days, renewing each day the Decoction.*

Perhaps surprisingly, the best cure for this malady was thought to be sexual intercourse. John Pechey explained that 'When the Disease is small, and chiefly arises from Obstructions of the Veins of the Womb, it is easily cured by Marriage in Young Virgins.' But Rivière cautioned that this was only the case if 'it could be legally done'. Of course, since this could only legitimately happen between married couples, medical texts recommended marriage as the cure. The sex cure was very well-known, and an anonymous ballad published in 1682 called *A Remedy for Greensickness* satirised a libidinous young woman who was lying on her bed hoping that a 'lusty lad' would appear to 'relieve me of my pain'. Luckily for her, the young man in the next room heard her sighs, and the climax of the ballad is that, having had sex once, the young woman remained unconvinced that she had been completely cured and wanted to have another 'bout' just to make sure. The 1662 edition of Nicholas Culpeper's *A Directory for Midwives* explained why sex was a reasonable cure:

> *It is probable, and agreeable to reason and experience that Venery is good. Hippocrates bids them presently marry, for if they conceive they are cured. Venery heats the womb and the parts adjacent, opens and loosens the passages, so that the terms may better flow to the womb.*

Culpeper did sound a note of caution however, and explained that if the disease was inveterate, 'there be a great Cacochymy' or humoral imbalance, then the healer needed to 'take that away before she be married'. Jane Sharp used Culpeper's book as the basis for some of the passages in her own midwifery guide and so reiterated this point but explained how important it was to remove the cachexy, because she had personally 'known some that have been so far from being cured, that they died by it; perhaps sooner than they would have done otherwise.' In other words, intercourse had worked too well and apparently caused the corruption to flood the woman's body resulting in her death.

From the mid-seventeenth century Thomas Sydenham was treating women with an iron supplement. His work, *The Complete Method of Curing almost all Diseases,* was only translated into English from Latin in 1694 however. This text claimed that many diseases in women 'naturally yield' to steel-based treatments. In greensickness:

> let the Patient take the Chalybeate Pills or Powder [...], more or less, according to her Age, drinking after them a Draught of any sort of Wine that pleaseth her, or of the corroborating Infusion of the Roots of Angelica there described. If she be not very weak, purge her once or twice, before she enter into this Course.

This idea explains why drinking the iron-rich chalybeate waters in spa towns was often seen as a good remedy for sufferers who had the means to make such a trip. The treatment was evidently well known, and a poem by John Wilmot, Earl of Rochester, dated 30 June 1675, and posthumously published by Matthew Prior in 1697 amongst others, mocked the clientele of the spa at Tunbridge Wells. In the poem, a mother has brought her daughter suffering from the 'headaches, pangs, and throes' of greensickness, and who is 'full sixteen, and never yet had *those*'. The woman's new friend rather crudely advises her to have her daughter married instead of relying on the waters:

> Get her a husband, madam:
> I married at that age, and never had 'em,
> Was just like her. Steel waters let alone;
> A back of steel will bring 'em better down.

While greensickness was very much in vogue in the period covered by this book, it is no longer a disease that is recognised medically, and from the 1920s, several essays were published claiming it no longer existed, including W. M. Fowler's, '*Chlorosis*: An *Obituary*' (1936). It might be the case that diagnoses of anorexia are preferred for a very similar set of symptoms, so this illness is a very good example of how diseases can be culturally determined.

Chapter 20

The Whites: A Most Troublesome Disease

'Ursula: "I do water the ground in knots, as I go, like a great Garden-pot"'
– Ben Jonson

As was discussed in the Introduction, the womb was repeatedly described as being the 'cause of six hundred miseries, and innumerable Calamities.' One of these many miseries was a disease often known simply as 'the whites'. Physicians used the Latin translation of this, *Fluor albus* (white flow), in their case notes. However, by the beginning of the eighteenth century, medics had begun to prefer the term still in use now, 'leucorrhoea' which has the same meaning but is Greek in origin; this mirrors a change in the way medics began to prefer the Greek term 'catamenia' for menstruation over the Latin form *menses* over the same time period. Leucorrhoea is the name now given for non-specific vaginal discharges.

The disease was so well known that it carried a number of other alternative names too. The book *The Practice of Physick* (1655) described how 'A Woman is said to have the Whites, the Woman's Flux, the Flux of the Womb, or the White Menstruals; when Exrementious Humours do flow from her Womb.' The white menstruals is a suggestive term that highlights the conception of this disease as similar to menstruation and accounts for other circumlocutions such as the one used by the sixteenth-century physician Thomas Raynalde who called it, the 'white flowers' in his 1545 edition of *The Birth of Mankind, otherwise named the Woman's Book*, or John Sadler in *The Sick Woman's Private Looking Glass* (1636), who called it the 'false courses.' Both courses and flowers were common names for menstrual periods routinely used in everyday speech.

The characteristics of this disease were discussed in the 1662 edition of *Culpeper's Directory for Midwives: or, A Guide for Women*. Culpeper was typically dramatic, suggesting that it was 'a foul excretion from the womb, white, and sometimes blue, or green, or reddish'. The symptoms appeared not 'at a set time, nor every month, but disorderly, longer or shorter. Before or after the Terms [terms being yet another synonym for periods] and when they are stopped.' This description implies that the disease resisted being confined to its nominative value, as it did not always present as a white flow.

Rivière's book described the unruly nature of the flow and said that these 'Excrementitious Humours do flow from her womb, either continually, or at least without any certain order, or course of time observed in their flowing.' Some women were thought to be more susceptible to this condition than others. An anonymous text by 'A Physician' from 1716, called *A Rational Account of the Natural Weakness of Women* explained that 'this illness is mostly occasioned by foregoing Distempers (tho' sometimes by sudden frights, violent Exercise, immoderate Venery, &c.).' In other words, women who were run-down by other recent illnesses, or perhaps a difficult delivery, might well develop the whites. Tellingly, this physician also added that too much exercise or sexual intercourse could also bring it on. However, when the midwife Jane Sharp wrote about this disease in 1671, she moderated these hyperbolic statements by observing that 'many have had this Disease long, and found no great hurt.' Most texts agreed that backache was the most certain sign of the whites. Eighteenth-century physician William Forster concurred. His book *A Treatise on the Causes of most Diseases* (1746) reported that:

> *You need only see a Woman's face to know if they are troubled with the Whites; for their Eyes have leaden Circles about them; their Cheeks are pale and Earth colour'd; they are every now and then clapping their Hands to their Back, which is a secret Confession they feel somewhat troublesome there, and such Women seldom fail of having Pain in their Backs.*

One interesting aspect of the disease though is that because medical writers thought it was so commonplace, they made references to it in chapters about all manner of other conditions without pausing to explain the term to their readers.

Secret Confessions: Diagnosis and Prognosis

In terms of diagnosing this condition, the disease was signified by more than just the flow itself and backache. John Sadler explained that patients presenting with this disease were characterised by such symptoms as: 'extentuation [emaciation] of the body, shortness and stinking of the breath, loathing of meat, pain in the head, swelling of the eyes and feet, melancholy [sadness].' If untreated, the prognosis was rather bleak. Another, more sensationalist text, *An Account of the Causes of some Particular Rebellious Distempers* (1670), claimed that 'if the Whites be neglected or not timely cured, they will bring great pain and weakness in the Back and whole Body, and occasion many other dangerous Maladies, as Cachexies [imbalanced humours], Dropsies, Consumptions, &c, which may prove fatal.' There was no end of medical texts picking up on this warning. The anonymous text by 'A Physician', which drew heavily on the 1670 text just cited, similarly warned that unless the whites was 'timely remedied, it certainly causes incurable Barrenness, and the Blood and Juices become more and more depauperated [thin, weak], till a deplorable Consumption, or Dropsy &c. ushers in Death to end the melancholy Tragedy.'

Confusion with Venereal Disease

Doctors believed that women were reluctant to consult them about this condition, perhaps in part because of the association with having had 'immoderate Venery' as the Physician mentioned above claimed. Another reason women might have been reluctant to go to their doctor until they were in great distress, and even perhaps thought in real danger of dying, was a worry that the physician might think that she had contracted a sexually transmitted disease instead. The main way doctors distinguished 'the whites' from a sexually transmitted discharge was that the flow associated with whites was meant to stop for the duration of a menstrual period, whereas gonorrhoea did not. Physician William Cockburn devoted a whole chapter in his 1715 book *The Symptoms, Nature, Cause, and Cure of Gonorrhoea* to an attempt to establish the differences between *fluor albus* and gonorrhoea. He stated that:

> *The next Difficulty that remains to be explained, is to find out the Difference between the* Fluor Albus *in Women and their Gonorrhoea: As also, by what Marks they may be known, since hitherto such Signs, as can show this difference, are still wanting. For the Humour that flows in the Whites is* Thick, White, Yellow, *and sometimes* Green, *often exciting a* Heat *of Urine: All which, being Symptoms of the Running of a Gonorrhoea, make the Characteristic of the Whites more hardly to be found.*

Cockburn was unconvinced by the widely held view that the whites stopped when a woman was menstruating. In fact, he rejected the argument altogether and insisted that 'this observation is really feigned, and altogether inconsistent with experience, and the Nature of the thing, it does not require our further Consideration.'

The potential for a conflation between the whites and venereal disease also had another implication: vulnerable women might be tempted to seek help from mountebanks and other quack healers rather than risk being embarrassed at the doctor's. Indeed, Cockburn suggested that women might have been encouraged to think that they might have a sexually transmitted disease and so 'upon this Appearance mercenary Clap-curers leave Women to be helped by the proper Methods of that Disease, exacting their Reward of having cured the Gonorrhoea.' This disturbing account implies that vulnerable and sick women were easy prey for quack-healers with unscrupulous practices. Cockburn was clearly alert to the abuse of women in this way when he noted that the reverse has never been heard of: a man with venereal discharges had never been diagnosed with the whites.

Of course the opposite was also true and women with venereal diseases might be diagnosed with the whites. In one incident noted by physician John Marten in his book on venereal disease, he claimed he had had to step in and cure a woman of a:

> Venereal Running, *which she got from her Husband, and had been for Cure in the Hands of one of the Quacks aforementioned, who telling her 'twas only the* Whites, *gave her astringents which stopped it, and told her she was well, she believed the same, and paid him three pounds for doing it.*

Marten himself, however, was often referred to as a quack, so was casting himself in the role of the experienced practitioner, who saved a woman from a disease which, he wrote, would otherwise have led 'to her Ruin.' Three pounds is itself a scandalously large sum to have charged, and so demonstrates the lengths a woman might have gone to, to achieve a cure for her vaginal discharges. These episodes also suggest that this apparent confusion, whereby vulnerable people were conned by profiteering medics who saw women as easy targets, did mean that prostitutes who had contracted a venereal disease could, as Marten put it 'cover their Whoredom with a pretence that it is the *Whites*'.

First Observe a Strict Diet: Treatment

The whites were commonly believed to be the result of a humoral imbalance within the woman's body. Midwife Jane Sharp even named her chapter on this disease, 'the Whites or Woman's disease, from corruption of Humours.'

William Cockburn explained that 'The Effects and causes [of the whites] are within a Woman herself' whereas he said, 'the Gonorrhoea is produced by Causes extrinsical [sic] to her', which is to say that the whites are caused by an internal humoral imbalance, caused for many reasons, but gonorrhoea is a disease which is contracted by external contact. Jane Sharp advised that 'To cure it, first observe a strict Diet; cleanse the whole body by purging; letting blood, Sweating, and Diuretics.' This regime was designed to dry out a body that was too wet, thus causing the excess humours to leak from the womb.

Women's handwritten manuscript books are filled with cures for this condition, which centre upon drying or purging the body. The books deal with this disease in lists alongside other diseases without the excitement and hyperbole of some of the more sensational medical texts, which implies that the condition was well known and was one for which a range of homemade cures were practised in a matter-of-fact way. Similarly, the case notes of John Hall contain an account of a patient suffering from the post-partum whites:

> *Mrs. Harvey, now Lady, very religious, five weeks after Child birth, was vexed with a great Flux of Whites, as also Pain and Weakness of the Back, was thus cured: Rx* [prescribed] *Dates as many as you please, cut them small, and with purified Honey make an Electuary. This she used in the morning. By this only Remedy she was cured, freed from her Pain which came often, stayed the Whites, and made her fat.*

Lady Harvey's symptoms included the ubiquitous backache as well as the discharge. Hall hoped this remedy would rebalance the body with a gentle laxative action. Hall's comment that Lady Harvey was inclined to religion might have been designed to offset any suggestion that she had contracted the disease from immoderate behaviour. It is an indication of how prevalent the condition was thought to be that William Forster advocated a preventative treatment which all women should routinely use: 'Repeated use of Cloves would defend many young Women from the Whites, which is a Misfortune many Women of all Ages are subject to, and which they might either prevent or cure by insisting on this Drug.'

As we will see throughout this section, there is great overlap between reproductive disorders. Both the pox and the whites could be confused with one another, and when applied to women both were a catchall name for various vaginal discharges. While some women, no doubt, had thrush infections, some of cases of the whites would, of course, be the normal lubrications of a healthy vagina.

Chapter 21

Infertility: A Defect in the Seed

'Nor fruitful showers your barren tops bestrew,
Nor fields of offerings ever on you grow'
– Anne Bradstreet

Bearing children in the early modern era was intrinsically connected to people's faith and their understanding of social roles and responsibilities. The Bible instructed men and women to be fruitful and populate the earth. This was emphasised more in the post-Reformation era, when the idolising of virginity in the figure of Mary was replaced by ideals about marriage. Bearing children also produced new souls to fill God's Church. Moreover, domestic harmony was, in part, reliant upon man and wife paying each other 'due benevolence', which was revealed through pregnancy. Although women's identities weren't solely constructed around maternity, since their work could also be central to their identity, for many women bearing children was an important social marker. It gave them authority and allowed them to participate in the shared culture of married women. Lady Margaret Hoby would regularly spend the day fasting and in private prayer, as she did on 7 October 1603, hoping that this would incline God to give her 'that blessing which I yet want' – a child. Lady Hoby was on her third marriage by this time and had no children. As a noblewoman she was obliged to provide healthcare to her 'family' of servants and other workers and in the course of this, delivered babies. This must have been poignant for a woman who wanted children as she did. Some who were unable to bear children were scorned and ridiculed by their neighbours, who made snide remarks or jeered at them in an argument. For men, being childless could be equally distressing and could have an impact on a man's reputation. Barrenness was thus not only a medical condition, but a social state.

Samuel Pepys, whilst at a party on 25 July 1664 to celebrate the birth of Anthony Joyce's newborn baby, asked the assembled women if they had any advice about his 'not getting of children'. Elizabeth and Samuel had been married for over eight years at this point and he was ever hopeful that they might conceive – his very first diary entry in 1660 described the couple's recent dashed hopes that Elizabeth was pregnant, and how the onset of her period had thus upset them both. The women happily obliged him and recommended drinking the juice of sage, or eating toast with tent (a type of red Spanish wine). These suggestions were not successful for the couple and they remained childless. He was not alone in dealing with this particular struggle; it is evident that many people had difficulties conceiving. One handwritten remedy collection belonging to Lady Ayscough included a note next to one remedy, designed to cleanse the reproductive system and make it ready for conception, that it had helped a Mrs Hone, who had been married for four years without conceiving a child. Sir Simonds d'Ewes, whose correspondence was published in the nineteenth century, recorded of his own birth that it was a great relief to his family because his mother had 'remained barren about six years after her marriage.'

Medical literature from the era explained in detail that there were many causes of infertility. A great many of the problems, deficiencies, and disorders that could result in barrenness were thought to affect women, and many medical writers blamed women, either explicitly or implicitly, for a couple's infertility. Daniel Sennert's *Practical Physick*, for example, claimed that 'Hence we may gather, that Barrenness is oftener from a fault in the women then the men.' This reasoning was based on the fact, as Sennert saw it, that men only needed to provide seed to conception, but women had to produce seed, retain the foetus, and nourish it. In many manuscript collections, remedies for barrenness were similarly aimed at female patients.

A key medical debate of this era affected how people thought about fertility. This was the argument over what reproductive material men and women contributed to conception. For some, both men and women produced 'seed' (seminal matter) that mixed in the womb to become a foetus that was nourished by menstrual blood. Advocates of this framework noted that women's bodies contained testicles (the ovaries), and that God made nothing in vain. Logically, therefore, women's testicles had to produce seed, in the same way that men's did. Importantly though, proponents of this model distinguished between men's seed – which sparked new life and imparted a soul to the offspring – and women's seed – which was cooler and less important than men's. Alternatively, some people believed that women did not produce seed, and that instead, conception occurred when a man's seed shaped and formed a woman's menstrual blood into a foetus. This theory frequently made use of an agricultural field and seed metaphor: the man planted his seed in the woman's soil; alternatively they used the agent and patient metaphor in which the male was the active agent. What model a medical writer, or patient, followed would change the potential range of causes of infertility. For the former, both men and women could be producing deficient seed, while a woman could also be producing deficient menstrual blood or could have a faulty womb; so, for example, sixteenth-century physician Thomas Raynalde pointed out in his 1545 reproduction guide, *The Birth of Mankind*, that a defect in any of the three factors could cause infertility. In the latter model faulty seed was restricted to the male body.

While it was accepted that women's bodies were colder and wetter than men's, being too cold or too wet meant women were thought unlikely to conceive. This is the reason prostitutes were assumed not to get pregnant in the course of their work. The abundance of semen collected in their bodies meant their wombs were too moist and slippery to retain the seed. As the prostitute Cornelia, in the anonymously authored erotic novel *The London Jilt* put it:

> *My Territory was so frequently cultivated by Five men, and that by this Reason it seemed there could not arise any Fruit, by Reason that I figured to myself that the too great abundance of Humidity would be capable of stifling it in its Birth.*

However, Cornelia's faith in contraception through multiple lovers was misplaced and after six months she found she was indeed pregnant. The humidity and slipperiness of the womb was the reason that women with leucorrhoea (the whites, a non-specific vaginal discharge, see Chapter 20) were also thought to be infertile.

While it could be a problem with the woman that meant a couple didn't conceive, medical texts reveal that popular assumptions that women were always blamed for infertility – often citing Henry VIII's attitudes to his many wives – are not strictly speaking true. In 1686 William Salmon noted that continual reproductive disappointments would lead to couples quarrelling about whom was to blame for their condition. Moreover, many medical texts included tests to establish which partner was sterile. These, of course, would not have been necessary if it was always believed to be the woman's fault. Most fertility tests required the man and the woman to urinate on a plant, usually wheat, barley, or corn. If the plant grew it was a sign that the party was fertile. Alternatively, each person urinated on a lettuce leaf; the urine that evaporated first identified whose body was barren. More than this, Nicholas Culpeper's translation of French physician Lazare Rivière's treatise went so far as to warn healers to 'diligently consider and inquire, whether Conception and Generation be not hindered by fault of the Man, or any deficiency in him. For in such a Case, It were vainly done to torment the Woman with a multitude of Medicines.'

As there were many causes of barrenness, including deficient production of seed, physical abnormalities of the reproductive organs, a lack of bodily heat – necessary for arousal, and any number of diseases that had a damaging effect on the reproductive body, there were many suggested remedies. There were, however, several popular options. Following the example of Mary of Modena, Catherine of Braganza, and other royal women suffering from fertility problems, those with the financial freedom to do so often frequented the baths in order to improve their fecundity. Robert Pierce, a Fellow of the Royal College of Physicians and medical practitioner in Bath, published his *Bath Memoirs* in 1697. This was promotional material for his services and so the wonderful efficacy of the cures should be taken with a pinch of salt, but Pierce was adamant that the baths had cured several women of inveterate barrenness. He wrote of a Mrs Hawkins from Marlborough, who had struggled to conceive for thirteen or fourteen years; and Lord Blessington's wife, 'a very weakly and sickly Person, having been some Years married, and never had a child.' In the poem 'Tunbridge Wells', mentioned in a previous chapter, John Wilmot, the Earl of Rochester, featured one woman who was patronising the spa who complained to her friend that 'We have a good estate, but have no child, / And I'm informed these wells will make a barren / Woman as fruitful as a coney [rabbit] warren.'

Barrenness did not only mean a struggle to conceive after marriage. Barrenness was also a temporary condition that could develop after the birth of several children. In the Tunbridge Wells poem, the mother of the teenage girl with greensickness was herself seeking a cure for secondary infertility, as it is known, having only had one daughter and no sons, to her husband's dismay. Robert Pierce noted that he had also cured several women suffering in this way, including a Mrs Clement who:

> had been a *Mother of Children*, but was so unhappy as to see them all buried; and after Nine Years ceasing to conceive with Child, and giving over the Hopes of it; being afflicted with Rheumatic Pains, *came to the Bath, in the year 87* [...] *She followed her bathing diligently, for a Month or Five Weeks, (till she found Ease of her Pains) then returned home; and tho' she had so long intermitted*

being pregnant, and despaired of ever being again a Mother, yet, in
a little time, she conceived with Child, and had, at her due time, two
Boys at a Birth.

Many cases of infertility must have resolved naturally, regardless of the medical interventions. For others, like Lady Hoby and Elizabeth Pepys, it seems it just wasn't meant to be and they had to come to terms with the fact that they would not bear children.

Chapter 22

False Conceptions and Miscarriages:
Breeding Moles

'Oh, Mr. Mooncalf, are you there? Prithee depart,
for I am very busy at present'

– Thomas Middleton

I n a diary entry from 1727, which served as a review of his year, James Clegg, a doctor from Derbyshire, described how his wife had been so poorly that May with a fever that she had been 'very near death'. The fever occurred in the immediate aftermath of her having delivered a 'false conception'. The episode left Ann infirm and with on-going lameness, and after having had nine children between 1705 and 1724, she had no further babies. An incidence of a false pregnancy was generally accepted to be a dangerous time for a woman. Gentleman William Coe noted in his diary for 11 July 1706 that: 'about midnight my wife had a false conception came from her, and was in great danger, but I thank God she grew very well in a few days.'

Several years after his wife's experience of a false pregnancy, Clegg treated a patient with the same condition. His diary entry for May 1731 relates the day that Mrs Waterhouse brought her daughter, Mrs White, for a consultation, fearing that she was suffering from bladder stones, or a 'fit of the gravel'. It became apparent that she was having labour pains and she soon delivered a 'small child of three months growth', with the aid of the midwife Clegg had summoned, but the next morning she also delivered a 'mole or false conception'. Mrs White's miscarriage was put down to a fright she had received when she had been set upon in Chesterfield. Frights were the most common explanation for a miscarriage but in Mrs White's case, the miscarriage seems to have been delayed until the foetus was decayed, and it was considered very fortunate that she had sought medical help such that she delivered these embryos while in a doctor's care. Clegg tended Mrs White through the night and the following day with balsam electuaries (a medicinal paste) and prayer – Clegg was a dissenting minister as well as a qualified physician – and the treatment seemed to provide some relief. Mr White came to visit his wife and stopped with the doctor and his family overnight, leaving Clegg with some '2 guineas for advice and attendance on his wife' who was well enough to leave for home some days later on the nineteenth.

Most of the reproduction guides published in this era included some discussion of the causes and treatments of false conceptions or molar pregnancies. The commonly agreed origin of the term 'mole' is from the Latin 'Molæ', a measure of weight, because moles were heavy. John Maubray's 1724 book, *The Female Physician Containing all the Diseases Incident to that Sex in Virgins, Wives and Widows*, noted that moles were like a 'millstone' for women. The amount of text space given to moles seems disproportionate to the probable incidence. Nowadays, the occurrence of a molar pregnancy has been put at around 1/1000 births; for unknown reasons, in less developed countries this statistic rises to 8/1000 births, and therefore, if it can be assumed that even if women in early modernity were at the higher end of the spectrum, a practitioner would not expect to see a 'true mole' more than once or twice in their career. The prime reason for this amount of coverage is probably because, first, this description was used by most texts as an almost catchall diagnosis, with the term 'false mole' mopping up any number of conditions, and, second, there was a huge cultural interest in apparent abnormalities or birth defects. In modern obstetrics, a molar pregnancy is thought to be caused by two possible events: first, a complete mole develops if the sperm fertilises an egg which has no nucleus, as the sperm then tries to duplicate itself to make up for the lack of genetic information, and a mass develops which resembles a bunch of grapes (hydatid vesicles). Second, and most frequently, two sperms might fertilize the same egg and the resultant growth might even contain a foetus, but one that will not develop to full term, which is known as is a partial mole. Seventeenth-century physician Percival Willughby, who wrote about it in his manuscript, 'Observations in Midwifery', told a story of a woman who experienced this:

> *I have had experience in a woman, which, lying very sick of a malignant fever, and being very weak, did suffer an abortion* [miscarriage]*; who, after the exclusion of the foetus, which was incorrupt, and entire, yet lay exceeding weak, with a disorderly pulse, in a cold sweat, as if she were a dying.*
>
> *I perceived the orifice of the womb was lax, soft, and very open, and her after purgings something noisome. Whereupon I suspected, that something did lurk in her womb, which did putrefy. And, putting in my hand, I extracted a false conception, as big as a goose egg which was*

made of a most thick, nervous, and, almost, gristly substance, having
some perforations in it, whereout did issue a viscid, putrefied matter, and
immediately, upon this, she was discharged of those grievous symptoms,
and suddenly, after, did perfectly recover.

At this time there were also said to be two main types of moles, but these distinctions do not equate to modern ones; there was a 'true mole' and a 'false mole'. There were also many sub-divisions of mole including 'windy' and 'watery' moles.

Early modern people also knew false conceptions as a moon-calf, which was because, in John Maubray's words, they 'frequently cast forth about the fourth *Month*'. 'Mooncalf' is explained by the *Oxford English Dictionary* as being '[f]ormerly regarded as being produced by the influence of the moon', and this is because the most common belief was that a mole was caused, like monsters were, by couples having intercourse during menstruation. It seems likely then that 'moon-calf' is a textual and cultural overhang from the theory that the moon somehow controlled women's menstrual cycles. The midwife Jane Sharp confirmed this, writing, 'without dispute, the principal cause is women's carnally knowing their Husbands, when their Terms [menstrual periods] are purging forth.' Thomas Chamberlayne's *The Complete Midwife's Practice* (1656), unusually, did not claim that intercourse while menstruating was the primary cause of a molar pregnancy, but explained that a weakness in the male seed might possibly be a cause. This view dates back centuries and was written in an English gynaecological guide from the fifteenth century based on the Trotula manuscripts, taken from the works of an eleventh century female physician. This manuscript stated that a 'true mola' occurred when the uterus retained the unfertilised woman's seed, for 'if it comes from a man's seed that is not powerful enough to be viable as a result of natural virtue and natural heat of the womb, in consequence, a lifeless, fleshy lump is produced'. *The Complete Midwife's Practice* also explained that a mole might be conceived when a 'woman lies with a great desire and lust with her husband, after she hath conceived, or when she hath retained her monthly courses beyond her time.' The best-selling guide to reproduction, *Aristotle's Masterpiece* (1684), agreed that moles could be caused by women being 'extremely Lascivious'. It is hard to imagine the pressure such ideas placed on women readers as, on the one hand it was thought imperative that they enjoyed sex, within marriage of course, and reached orgasm to conceive, but yet they should not be too lascivious and risk endangering their reproductive health.

Just as was the case with scurvy, 'mooncalf' was also used pejoratively as an insult to describe a fickle person or even to mock a bad idea.

False Moles

The Complete Midwife's Practice explained that the false-mole could be a 'windy mole' caused by 'the weak heat of the matrix [womb]' and adjacent organs such as the liver and spleen; alternatively the mole might be a 'watery mole' which was caused by the liver's failure to assimilate 'the blood which is sent thither'; the 'humorous mole' was thought to be formed from a collection of corrupt humours in the womb, including the 'whites [leucorrhoea], or certain watery purgations which sweat forth from the menstrous veins' – the veins which supplied blood to the womb and from where menstrual periods were thought to flow; a 'membranous mole' was a 'skin or bag, which is garnished with many white and transparent vessels'; finally, there was the possibility of a pendant mole, which was a 'piece of flesh, hanging within the inner neck.' In modern gynaecology, many of the symptoms that led to a diagnosis of a false mole would have other explanations. For example, Jane Sharp noted that 'many aged women live many years with a Mole in the body, yet it never stinks nor corrupts though they keep them till they die', and this would probably now be considered to indicate it was a fibroid or benign tumour in the womb.

Symptoms and Treatments

In *The Sick Woman's Private Looking Glass* (1636), John Sadler described how to diagnose a molar pregnancy: 'the signs of a mole are these. The months [periods] are suppressed the appetite is depraved, the breasts swell, and the belly is puffed up and waxeth hard.' The difficulty was, as Sadler admitted, 'Thus far the signs of a breeding woman, and of one that beareth a mole are all one.' The distinction, he claimed, 'is taken from the motion of a mole; it may be felt to move in the womb before the third month, which the infant cannot.' Sadler explained that this sensation of movement was caused by the 'faculty of the womb', not through 'the intelligent power of the mole', because the mole 'lives not a life animal, but [lives] in the manner of a plant.' The second sign was that 'in a mole, the belly is suddenly puffed up', and thirdly: 'the belly being pressed with the hand, the mole gives way, and the hand being taken away it returns to the place again.' Finally and most alarmingly, Sadler explained that, 'the childe continues in the womb not above eleven months; but a mole continues sometimes four or five years.'

Most medical writers urged a gentle approach to the treatment of a suspected molar pregnancy. Indeed, Willughby recommended that the matter was left to nature as far as possible as she made the best midwife in this situation. He went further, stating 'let not the midwife trouble the woman in being too busy, with her too much officiousness, to bring it away, for that nature, and her own strength, with quiet keeping, and comfortable warmness, will soonest free her of these sufferings.'

In 1695 Bernard Smith wrote to Edward Clarke about his wife Mary's miscarriage, and described the treatment he had given her, which included a cordial made of ground pearls for her vomiting. Again his treatment focused on the after-effects of the event, not direct intervention. He went on to reassure Clarke that 'there was no [child] but a false conception which much of [noisily] came off'. Perhaps the widespread belief in moles and false pregnancies provided comfort to some couples who could more easily accept the loss of a false pregnancy than a potential baby.

Faking a False Pregnancy

At least one woman used common knowledge about moles to procure an abortion according to a story recounted by Percival Willughby. He was considering the question of whether the cervix could be artificially opened during pregnancy and concluded that it could because of the following anecdote communicated to him by 'a real, true friend':

> *Coming from Gloucester, in my returning homeward to Derby, I met with a good friend, a Dr of Physick, and a practicer in midwifery. He certified me, that he was entreated, by a Gentlewoman, to afford her his help, and assistance; for that she knew, that there was a false conception in her womb, which would be her ruin, unless, by his skill, he could open the womb, and take it forth.*
>
> *He was over persuaded by her, giving credence unto her words, and being entreated to try his skill, and to use the utmost of his endeavours, to perform this work; he slid up his hands, and forced the orifice of the womb with his finger end, moving, and thrusting it gently, for a reasonable space, against the orifice of the womb. After some time, by these ways, and her enforcements, the womb was opened, and, forthwith, the waters flowed; and, within a short space after, the birth of a child followed.*

To the doctor's mortification he had delivered a premature baby not a mole, and 'At the sight thereof he was much troubled (he told it to me with a great deal of sorrow) and said unto her, that he was displeased with her evil doings. But she made slight of his rebukes, and words.' The woman was from a prominent family of great esteem, and so the physician left her name out of his tale for the sake of their reputation. It seems likely that this duplicity had a hand in the unnamed gentlewoman's eventual demise as her practice of consulting several physicians at once, without the others' knowledge, 'to cover her lewdness' caused her to take conflicting medications resulting in her death by 'physick'.

Miscarriages

It was not just false conceptions that ended in miscarriage, women could miscarry for all manner of reasons, and often for causes unknown. Unfortunately, miscarriages were not uncommon and were discussed regularly in medical literature, diaries, and correspondence. That they were a feature of many women's reproductive lives did not, though, diminish the anxiety and fear women experienced when faced with the loss of their child, nor did it diminish the anguish of miscarrying.

Women's fears about the potential for a miscarriage were perhaps not allayed by the information presented in medical texts. Authors explained that several internal factors could threaten the foetus: the initial conception might be too weak to survive, the child might lack nourishment in the womb, or might be squashed and constricted by a small womb. More than this though, authors throughout the sixteenth, seventeenth and eighteenth centuries explained to women that a plethora of illness, actions, and emotions could jeopardise a pregnancy, as was discussed in the smallpox chapter, for example. Jane Sharp claimed in her *Midwives Book* that 'There are abundance of causes whereby women are driven to abort, or miscarry.' These causes included inflammations, fainting, vomiting, sneezing, coughing, violent motions (such as running or dancing), receiving blows to the stomach or back, and excessive passions – sadness, fear, anger and sorrow. Alessandro Massaria's *Woman's Counsellor* (1657), summarised that 'It oftentimes comes to pass with women with child, as with the fruit upon a Tree; which being young and tender, hangs on brittle stalks, and is easily blown off with every wind'.

Men were attuned to the potential for bouts of ill health to cause a miscarriage. Sir Arthur Kaye wrote to 'Dear Sister Wilmot' explaining that he feared his wife might have a miscarriage, but that she came through the danger: 'for though she was from Monday last to Friday extremely ill, yet she then overcame the hazardous symptoms that justly alarmed us, & I thank God is now much better.' Likewise the Earl of Halifax wrote to the Bishop John Moore in Ely describing his wife's fever. He revealed that this had caused him to worry that she might lose her baby: 'She has yet no signs of miscarrying but in her condition, I am under all the apprehensions Imaginable for her'.

Popular literature also played on the idea that pregnancy, particularly early pregnancy, was precarious. A. Marsh's 1682 satirical piece, the *Ten Pleasures of Marriage*, hinted that husbands had to walk on eggshells around wives who struggled to conceive and carry a foetus to term because emotional upset could cause a miscarriage. He wrote, 'he dares not anger her or give her a sour countenance; fearing that if she might have conceived, that would be the means of turning the tide.' If the worst happened, medical texts warned that the onset of a miscarriage would be marked by physical signs, the breasts would sag, the woman would experience great pain and the body would shake and tremble.

Not only was miscarriage an emotional time for women, it posed a considerable threat to their health. Anna, Lady Meautys, wrote to Jane, Lady Cornwallis Bacon, in March 1641 explaining the perilous state she had been in after miscarrying. She wrote:

> *Now concerning myself, since the departure of my daughter I have been very dangerously ill. I was gone with child three months, at the end of which time I did miscarry and was in that extremity that those that were about me did not think I should have escaped, and for one particular I had no hope for this life.*

Preventing Miscarriages

Those who knew that they were liable to suffer from a miscarriage were encouraged to take medical precautions before they fell pregnant. Nicholas Culpeper's text advised, 'remove the causes of weakness, and strengthen it. Use things that strengthen the womb and child.' People also resorted to a range of bodily adornments, like charms, which through their occult qualities protected the pregnancy. Importantly though, such items had to be worn above the midriff; if they were worn below the belly, their qualities would work in the opposite way and might provoke birth. John Locke recorded in

1682 that 'Our Lady's nut is a most approved remedy against miscarriages if worn above the middle next the skin, if below it helps delivery.' This remedy he had gained from Mr Thistlethwaite. The most common of these charms was the 'eagle stone', a hollow stone in which a smaller stone resided that rattled when shaken. This stone and its safely encased pebble mirrored the pregnant body. Like other charms, it was meant to be bound to the left arm throughout pregnancy to prevent miscarriage, and was then moved during labour to assist the birth. Not everyone was convinced that such things helped, but there was clearly some willingness to believe that they would. In 1725 one agitated father, H. Peatt, wrote to the royal physician Sir Hans Sloane asking 'pray Sir do you think an Eagle Stone of any use to prevent miscarrying?'

If these measures failed and the signs of an impending miscarriage appeared, medical texts advised women to use astringents which would close the vagina, thus keeping a pregnancy inside the body. These books were filled with remedies with titles like 'to hinder Abortion' or 'to prevent miscarriage'. The recipe book attributed to Elizabeth Okeover offered several suggestions for women in this unenviable position. For example, 'In danger of miscarriage' a woman should take cinnamon comfit and put it into syrup of althea (a genus of plants including marsh mallows and hollyhock), and eat them after they had had time to absorb the oil. A more complex remedy in the manuscript invited women to lie down in a warm bed and: 'Drink a good drought of fair water'. This was followed by taking 3oz of ale with scarlet or purple silk shredded very small, the 'treads' (possibly the round, white spot on the surface of the yolk, the germinal vesicle) of eighteen eggs, and conserve of red roses. This mixture was, it was recommended, taken for three mornings and three nights while the woman laid a piece of toast soaked in muscadine wine to the navel. Laying warm toast soaked in wine and spices to the stomach was a popular response. It was also recommended in the *Countryman's Physician* (1680): 'As soon as she perceives the least suspicion of miscarrying, apply to her naval a hot loaf new out of the oven cut in the middle, dipt in Malaga wine, sprinkled with powder of Cloves and Nutmegs, and bind it close on.' Jane Sharp wasn't convinced by the effectiveness of warm toast and said that bruised tansy in warm muscadine worked better.

As well as charms worn around the midriff, other types of girdles were also recommended. The recipe book attributed to Anne Brumwich suggested spreading suet upon a piece of white leather and sticking this to the belly with wax. The woman had to wear this 'continually' throughout the pregnancy. Anne's book also included remedies designed to ward off miscarriage commended by the Duchess of Devonshire, the Duchess of Buckingham, the Countess of Moulgrave, and Lord Chesterfield.

As Anna Meautys's letter and the discussion of false conception have shown, miscarriage was considered to be potentially life threatening. John Hall recorded that he had attended 28-year-old Joyce Broughton after she suffered a miscarriage in 1620. She suffered from vomiting, fainting and was 'in danger of Death'. Medical texts and remedy collections also attest to the perilous position women found themselves in after a miscarriage. Elizabeth Okeover's book included two remedies which had been prescribed to 'my sister' when she had suffered violent 'flux' – heavy bleeding – after a miscarriage. Yet despite this, whether a false conception, a mole, or any other kind of pregnancy was terminated in this way, the positive news is that then as now, most women would go on to experience healthy pregnancies subsequently.

Chapter 23

Venereal Disease: The French Pox,
a New Disease

*'The French Pox! Our Pox: S'blood we have them in as good
form as they man: what?'*

– Ben Jonson

T he vision of a pock marked and patched face is one that for many is synonymous with the early modern era. The rampant spread of the pox, its devastating effects on the skin, and its notoriously danger-ous treatment with mercury have rightly secured this contagious and fearful disease a place in the popular mind-set. The disease was rife, and in the later seventeenth century the sexual excesses associated with the high-living Restoration Court meant that it was endemic in royal circles. The 2006 film *The Libertine* starring Johnny Depp as John Wilmot, Earl of Rochester, depicts this well. In the popular imagination the pox is another name for syphilis. Yet early modern medical practitioners were not just talking about the syphilis, but gonorrhoea *and* syphilis. There were many names for this disease including the pox, 'a Clap', the French disease, the French pox, the *Morbus Gallicus*, and the *Lues Venerea*. The chemical physician Thomas O'Dowde also wrote that it was commonly called 'The Old Gentleman'.

Unlike many of the diseases early modern men and women encountered, the ancient Greek medical authorities had not extensively investigated and described the *Morbus Gallicus*. It was a new disease requiring investigation and innovation on the part of physicians and surgeons. In 1662 Richard Bunworth explained when the disease had first appeared in Western Europe:

> *The French Pox is certainly a new disease, and not known in Europe till within this hundred years: For when Charles the eight king of France besieged Naples, which was in the year 1494, it first began to spread itself, not only through his army, but through all Italy.*

That the disease had been spread by camp followers of the French army, who themselves had then spread the disease throughout Europe as they left the siege, was one, perhaps the most, popular understanding of where the disease had come from.

An alternative theory argued that pox had travelled with Columbus when he returned to Palos, Spain, from Hispaniola in 1493. His own son had written that when Columbus returned in 1498 he was gravely ill of the *Morbus Gallicus*, or the French Disease. Some writers combined the two theories, like Gideon Harvey who explained in his book *Little Venus Unmasked* (1670) that,

> Neapolitan Spaniards, *some of whom having been latterly abroad with Columbus, in the Year 1492, upon the discovery of the new World, or West Indies, after two Years absence, arrived back to their native Country* [...] *which they soon made present of to several of their dearest* Julietta's at Naples; *for immediately upon their arrival in Spain, they were hurried away to* Naples *to reinforce the Garrison.*

In this telling, Columbus's troops were the soldiers who spread the disease at Naples. Implicit in both of these descriptions though, were the women, predominantly prostitutes, who followed the camps to ply their trade and who facilitated the spread of the disease.

Sin and the Spread of the Disease

Wherever it came from, there were several theories about how and why the disease suddenly appeared. People quickly realised that the disease spread through sexual contact. This meant that just as quickly it was thought to be a punishment from God for lewd behaviour. Thomas O'Dowde, writing in his 1665 book *The Poor Man's Physician*, described how one of his patients, a 64-year-old man, had fallen 'under the sin of youth or folly of his age'. Another patient he described as a 'virtuous *Lady*', but was clear that she had caught the disease as a result of 'one night's kindness to a Friend'. Promiscuity and sexual indulgence were, therefore, considered to be the primary reasons why people ended up with the clap.

Most likely because of this association, medical books made attempts to suggest that people could catch the disease innocently. Authors like the eminent surgeon of St Bartholomew's hospital in London, William Clowes, claimed that simply sharing a bed with a 'pocky' person, or being in contact with their bedsheets, was enough to catch the disease. Likewise, some writers argued that the disease infected people who used the same close stool as a pox patient, or who shared drinking vessels and cups with the diseased, particularly if the victim had an ulcerous mouth. These suggestions were rather controversial. Not everyone accepted that the disease spread in this way, and some, like John Astruc, claimed in his treatise on the disease (1736, translated into English some years later) that 'it may be, that these were all fictions framed by the diseased to conceal their own naughtiness.'

Whores, Wet Nurses and Women

Medical textbooks blamed women for the spread of the disease in numerous ways. Because of their link to sexual immorality, prostitutes became an obvious target for vitriol. A seventeenth-century translation of Levinus Lemnius's *Secret Miracles* claimed that: 'This disease is taken from pocky sick people, and by lying with whores whose privities are infected with buboes.' In particular, medical men complained that prostitutes continued to ply their trade when infected and lied to potential clients, telling them they were free of the disease, and tricking them into unsafe sex.

More than this though, as the period progressed, more and more medical writers suggested that the disease could be 'bred' or created inside a woman's womb. The mixing of the semen of multiple men inside overly hot wombs caused a putrefaction. The seeds 'degenerated into a high malignancy', or disease. Prostitutes were thus a prime target because their wombs often contained the semen of different men. Moreover, because of their continual engagement in sexual activity, as the humoral model suggested, their bodies, and importantly their wombs, were more heated than ordinary women. But not all medical texts specified that this process occurred in the wombs of prostitutes. Promiscuous women who heated their bodies with repeated sexual encounters were just as likely to end up creating the disease. Historian Kevin Siena has called this the 'putrefaction theory' and argued that, as it took hold of the popular mind-set, it provided a way of suggesting that all women were *potential* harbingers of the disease – any woman had the capacity to mix and heat the seeds of numerous men, and so any woman could be a potential threat. In adopting these ideas the early modern populace had medical backing for their pre-existing ideas about women's modesty, and the dangers of female promiscuity and sexual desire.

In one rather unique text, *The Surgeon's Assistant* (1703), John Browne even claimed that beautiful women were more likely to catch the disease, and then pass it to someone else, than ugly women. This was not only because he believed ugly women were less likely to secure sexual partners. Medical theory postulated that desire stimulated the body's natural heat. Browne therefore theorised that beautiful women would cause greater arousal in the men they slept with, increasing the chances that the encounter would result in infection. Conversely, having sex with an ugly woman offered some measure of protection against the disease because men's bodies wouldn't be heated as much by the flames of desire and so they were less likely to contract the pox. The seventeenth-century French medical writer Nicolas Venette, whose works were translated into English in the early eighteenth century and reprinted numerous times, corroborated Browne's theories on sexual desire claiming that 'ugliness calms all our Raptures; far from exciting us to Love, it rather make us to abhor all its Pleasure. If peradventrue we are obliged to approach an ugly Woman, our secret Parts slacken rather than stiffen'.

In line with these ideas about women, medical writings by physicians and surgeons adopted the rhetoric that it was women who spread the disease – rather than the men who slept with them. This was due, in part, to the way in which such texts often assumed that the reader was male. They thus addressed men to be careful of potential partners who might be carrying the disease, you couldn't be too careful. In his *Poor Man's Physician* (1665), Thomas O'Dowde told the story of a man he cured of 'a Clap' who was 'a good man of *London* having innocently (I mean from his Wife) got a Clap.' This tone had perhaps lessened in the eighteenth century, despite the increasing acceptance that all women might potentially be a source of contagion. John Marten, for example, wrote that 'we know it to be now a-days gotten for the most part by the impure and carnal Embrace of an infected Person', rather than an infected woman.

In addition to spreading the disease to male partners women's bodies were also blamed for children succumbing to the pox. It was known that children born to pocky parents were likely to have the disease. As John Marten rather simply stated 'the Child of an unclean Parent may bring the Distemper into the World with it.' Women and children were then bound together as agents of contagion. These poor children might pass the disease to a wet nurse during suckling. Marten recited the tale of one unfortunate woman who took a 2-month-old child to suckle. Very soon 'her breasts all over [had] spread with a Humour, beginning first at the Nipple, which swelled the Glands [...] before she so much as imagined what should be the Cause thereof.' Caught unawares the woman was luckily 'cured' by Marten's treatments. In an earlier anecdote, O'Dowde had noted that a patient came to consult him for a painfully ulcerated throat who also had 'half her *Uvula* seized, and three large and deep sores on her forehead, not being able to swallow or drink other than Broth [...] I assured her it was a Pox of the worst sort', to which the woman replied, 'it came on by suckling a Child'. O'Dowde rather sarcastically replied that he hoped it was a 'Man-Child', but while he didn't buy her story, he did agree to treat her.

Conversely it was common knowledge that 'pure' children received the disease from infected wet nurses and brought it back to their own families. Marten and others rebuked these women for their recklessness and greed. He claimed that some wet nurses wilfully deceived potential clients so that they did not miss out on work and earnings:

> it is great pity, poor innocent Babes [...] should be (as they too frequently are) deprived of their Lives, and at the best of their Healths, by the barbarous Treatment of their polluted Attendance; who though they too well know before-hand what Distempers they have upon them, will for the sake of the Money run the hazard of the Children's Lives.

He concluded that both parents and 'wholesome' wet nurses needed to be careful when selecting children, or nurses, because by injudicious selection 'many Families have been undone'.

Virulent and Corrosive Matter: Symptoms

Given its devastating symptoms it is unsurprising that medical writers expended considerable effort laying blame for the spread of the disease. Many different texts noted that the disease could manifest in different ways, depending on how the patient caught the infection and its severity. Yet despite suggestions that some pox was 'slighter' than others, none of the symptoms seem trivial. Gideon Harvey, for example, noted that the 'slightest sort' of the disease caused the hair of the head and beard to fall out. As the disease increased in severity the patient would suffer from red and yellow spots over the skin, that would gradually scab over and turn into foul running sores. Once buboes had developed, the disease would gradually corrupt the blood, the liver, and then the bones and sinews. This final stage caused the bones to become very painful. Numerous preserved syphilitic skulls reveal how painful this would have been and the disfiguring effects this corrosion of the bones could cause.

In addition to these torments patients might experience a 'gleet' – a shedding of matter from their genitals – burning sensations when urinating, genital warts, ulcers, fevers, and 'racking Night-Pains'. Parisian physician

Jean Fernel recorded how bad these symptoms could be, offering the example of one 32-year-old man who was so ulcerated that his clothes became stiff with the matter that oozed from his sores, and another 50-year-old patient who lost all of his toe nails. Robert Bayfield, writing in 1655, suggested that patients could lose their eyesight, that the eyelids could be corroded, that the nose might fall flat and that, in men, the penis could become gangrenous. The pox was therefore not only a painful and shameful disease, but one that could cause permanent deformities.

Although we might think it was easy to identify and self-diagnose the pox based purely on its symptoms, one domestic recipe collection suggests that this wasn't always the case. The author included 'A Plaster to know whether a sore be *Morbus Gallicum* or not.' The plaster was made from the fat of an adder, the fat of fresh beetles and butter, with turpentine and 'Romine'. The final ingredient was verdigris; once the ingredients were combined, the plaster was laid on the sore. If when the patient removed the plaster it was white, then the patient knew they were suffering from venereal disease. If, however, the verdigris had retained its former green colour, the patient was safe. The author offered no suggestion for how long the plaster took to change colour, so we might imagine a patient peeking at the colour and returning the plaster to the sore in the hopes that it might eventually change colour.

A Night with Venus a Lifetime with Mercury

Despite the complexity of the condition some medical writers were optimistic. The famous French surgeon Ambroise Paré, for example, claimed that the disease was now 'far more mild and easy to be cured than that which was in former times.' This would seem to offer hope and consolation to pox victims. But Paré noted that cures were time-sensitive. If the disease was newly caught and had few symptoms, and particularly if the patient was young and of good constitution, then he claimed the 'cure is easy'. However, if the disease was of long standing, had many symptoms, or was characterised by a continued pain in the head and rottenness of the bones, if the body was ulcerated or weak, then attempting a cure was entirely in vain and was likely to be ineffective.

Sellers of patent drugs for these conditions were also exceptionally optimistic given the circumstances. *The Common Sense or The Englishman's Journal* carried an advertisement in May 1742 that typified this overly optimistic outlook. The advert exclaimed 'Dr. Nelson's most wonderful Panacea for Confirmed Venereal Lues' cured patients 'easily, and insensibly'. The author claimed that the remedy was 'admired and recommended by all that have taken it.' More than being a sensational drug able to cure even those who had been brought low by repeated mercurial treatments, this particular drug was better, according to the author, because it was 'also exceeding pleasant to take, as well as delightful in its effects.' Advertisements were liable to exaggerate and so played up to patient-consumers' desires for efficacy. Nonetheless, they did send the message that the disease could be, and if they were to be believed, had been, cured.

There were two key treatment plans offered to early modern patients. The first of these was mercury or quicksilver. John Marten described this substance as follows:

> It is a Mineral so penetrating, that it is capable of entering through the Pores of the Skin into the Mass of Blood […] which it wonderfully dissolves and rarefies, making the Blood fluxile, freeing it from Stagnations, Obstructions, Scoring the Gland, &c.

This it could do because mercury was heavier than the blood and so had the momentum to break through any particle. In the sixteenth century, healers applied mercury externally through ointments, plasters and rubs; later in the era people consumed mercury internally and exposed themselves to mercury 'fumes' to induce sweating. In order to be fumigated, patients were seated in a confined and sealed space with the mercury so that the fumes would rise towards the body. Mercury treatment required a considerable time commitment, up to thirty days. This of course meant that relations, neighbours and acquaintances could identify pocky patients by their absence from normal life caused by lengthy treatment.

Those treated for venereal disease clearly valued their privacy. Richard Wiseman, sergeant surgeon to Charles II, explained that one of his patients got very annoyed when asked if his swollen groin was the result of venereal disease. The patient maintained that his condition was the result of excessive drinking and moved two miles away to avoid further discussions about the issue. Some managed to maintain some degree of secrecy. In 1739, Catherine Demay appeared at the Old Bailey charged with murdering Michael Dunn. It was alleged that she had put a quantity of cantharides (Spanish fly) in his coffee. Cantharides were used medicinally as an aphrodisiac and in venereal disease cases, and were a known poison. The court case therefore attempted to establish whether Michael had consumed the drug as a treatment for venereal disease. If he had done so, then he had managed to keep this relatively quiet. He told the doctors and apothecaries who treated him that he did not have the disease. Although one man – James Gilstrop – told the court that Michael had revealed to him that 'I have got the foul Distemper', and showed him a box of pills he was taking as a cure. Thankfully for Catherine there was enough doubt about whether Michael had been taking this dangerous drug as a remedy for the pox for her to be acquitted of the murder.

Quacks and sellers of patent medicines played on these desires and made it clear in their adverts that their cures were quick and secretive. In two early eighteenth-century pamphlets, *The Practical Scheme of Secret Injuries. And Broken Constitutions* (1719) and *The Secret Patient's Diary* (1725), the author attempted to entice potential customers by repeatedly stating that the medicines he provided offered a secret means for the embarrassed to hide their condition. Patients were able to purchase the remedies by letter without a medical consultation, and so didn't even need to reveal their problems to a physician. Likewise, the patients took their drugs while they continued their everyday life, it wasn't necessary to remain in a bedchamber to sweat or salivate.

It was not just isolation that could identify a patient undergoing mercurial treatments. Mercurial remedies were almost as bad as the disease, causing a range of significant deformities that were easily recognisable or, as happened to Michael Dunn, death. John Marten provided many tales of patients who died taking poorly prepared mercurial treatments. One example was 'A certain slovenly itchy Man, having all his Skin defiled with that Distemper, and his Body with Lice; did by the Advice of some simple Woman, smear one Night all his Chest with Quicksilver and Fasting-spittle mingled together. After which he laid himself down to Sleep and never awaked.'

Medical writers were aware that mercury was a dangerous substance for the body. Marten, for example, explained that Goldsmiths, mirror makers and others who dealt with quicksilver in their work were 'seldom healthful and long-lived'; rather, they were subject to numbness, trembling, palsy, convulsions, catarrhs, and apoplexy. Those who had received quicksilver medicines had suffered miscarriages, gone blind, lost their hearing or their sense of smell, had suffered lameness, spasms, and fallen into 'Raving and Madness'. Perhaps the most obvious sign of mercurial salivation gone wrong was the loss of the palate and collapse of the nose, which made people 'an Object of Pity' to those who saw them. Despite all of these concerns Marten was not against the use of mercury, but was clear that a skilled practitioner must use it judiciously.

An alternative to mercurial treatments was guaiacum, otherwise known as 'pock wood', 'holy wood' or *lignum vitae*. According to medical texts, the Spanish brought this new world remedy to Europe; while Customs and Excise books reveal that England was receiving imports of the wood from the late seventeenth century. Ulrich von Hutten's sixteenth-century book, *Of the Wood called Guaiacum,* outlined the provenance and use of the substance. He explained that for use in medicine the wood had to be made as small as possible, creating shavings, or a powder by grinding the wood in a mortar. After soaking overnight in water the wood was gently boiled until the mixture reduced by half. The scum that rose to the top of the vessel during this process was used to anoint pocky sores. The wood was then strained and seethed again with the second residue being given to patients to drink with their meat. This evidently might have been preferable to mercurial treatments and it remained popular into the eighteenth century. *The Lady's Companion* (1743) included the 'Raspings of Guaiacum' mixed with liquorish, rhubarb, salt of steel, beer, and salt of tartar, as a remedy for the venereal disease. Although popular, not everyone was convinced of guaiacum's efficacy. Ambroise Paré lamented that the wood did not have 'sufficient strength to extinguish the venom of the venerous virulency [sic], but only to give it ease for a time.'

A Frightful Vision

Given its devastating effects and ubiquity in early modernity, it is no wonder that the *Morbus Gallicus* captured the popular imagination. It turned pleasure into pain and revealed vividly to the world the consequences of sexual immorality. It was a frightful condition with a frightful treatment and little chance of long-term survival, as Hogarth depicted in his illustration series the Harlot's Progress (1731), where an elderly bawd coerces a fresh-faced young woman into prostitution on her arrival in London. The new prostitute soon ends up in Bridewell prison where she contracts, and dies from, venereal disease aged just 23. The story of the innocent country girl being corrupted when she arrived in the city was told in numerous fictional accounts, and ultimately in John Cleland's *The Memoirs of a Woman of Pleasure* (published in 1748, but written a couple of decades before). The fiction must have reflected the stories of many men and women, not just prostitutes, who found themselves ravaged by the disease. This is especially likely with a disease which can appear to go into remission, leaving the sufferer believing themselves cured by treatments such as mercury fumes, only to be still carrying it and passing it on.

Afterword

There was only space enough to explore a number of common conditions in this book. Other complaints such as apoplexy, consumption, impostumes (abscesses), quinsy, priapism, rickets, rising of the lights (chronic coughing), sciatica, and surfeit will have to wait for another time.

We began with Sarah Wigges's rhyme about living well and dying never, and the examples in the book show time and again how seriously early modern people took the task of maintaining their health, within a framework where disease and ill health were inextricably linked to a person's spiritual health too.

As well as women able to make up homemade cures in their kitchens, the numbers and range of professions involved in healthcare was significant. Most of these advocated increasing excretion through laxatives and emetics as the first line of treatment, effectively aiding the body to remove what ailed it. Despite the rise in chemical and mechanical theories, humoralism remained the standard against which other treatments were viewed and the Hippocratic model of balance remained key.

Along the way we have seen how people responded to their medical complaints and faced pain, discomfort and death with fortitude, optimism (often aided by prayer), and by taking the initiative. We have also seen how devastating and demoralising ill health could be. In amongst all of this the book has revealed some surprises, in particular the number of times earthworms were the suggested cure for ailments.

List of Illustrations

Unless otherwise stated, all images are reproduced courtesy of the Wellcome Library, London.

'Yellow choler, also known as bile (hence bilious): the hot and dry humour. People with this as their dominant humour were often thought to have a fiery temperament. It is linked to summer and to fire.'

'Blood, sanguine constitution: hot and moist humour associated with childhood, Spring and the element air.'

'Phlegm: Cold and moist, often associated with old age. It is linked to the element water and to the winter season.'

'Melancholy or Black Bile: Cold and Dry. Linked with Autumn and the earth.'

Ague

'Fever, represented as a frenzied beast, stands racked in the centre of a room, while a blue monster, representing ague, ensnares his victim by the fireside; a doctor writes prescriptions to the right, 1788.'

Dropsy

'Johann Gottfried Matthes (Mathes), a "natural healer", taking the pulse of a patient suffering from the dropsy, 1784.'

'A man suffering from dropsy dictating his will whilst a physician takes his pulse, he is surrounded by his wife and friend.'

Smallpox

'Portrait of Lady Mary Wortley Montague, whose early support for inoculation for smallpox pioneered the preventative method in the eighteenth century.'

Sight Problems

'The patient is held in place while an operation is performed on his eye, 1594.'

'Seventeenth-century eye-glasses with horn-rims and hinged metal bridge in cardboard case with initials "I.B."'

Gout

'James Gillray, "The Gout", 1799.'

'Two gout sufferers, the richer carried on a litter, the poorer using crutches; (background) a man being treated for gout, 1559.'

Headaches

'Portrait of Valentine Greatrakes laying on his hands. The window in the corner shows several successful "cures", c.1666.'

'One patient lies still as trepanning is performed on his skull. Another apprehensive-looking man sits beside him being prepared to undergo the same operation, 1594.'

Cancer

'Elizabeth Hopkins of Oxford, showing a breast with cancer which was removed by Sir William Read, 1700.'

Infestations

'A drawing of a flea from Robert Hooke's *Micrographia*, 1665.'

'Boy combing lice out of hair, 1639.'

Kidney and Bladder Stones

'Lithotomy (surgical removal of a stone or stones from the urinary tract) being performed, 1707.'

'Instruments used in a lithotomy, 1708.'

King's Evil

'Charles II touching a patient for the king's evil (scrofula) surrounded by courtiers, clergy and general public.'

Plague

'Bill of Mortality from August 15–22, 1665, at the height of the Great Plague.'

'Sixteenth-century pomander for protecting against the plague.' Image courtesy of the Rijksmuseum, Netherlands.

'Two physicians, one representing George Thompson, dissecting the corpse of a plague sufferer, from his book on the plague *Loimotomia; or the Pest Anatomized*, 1666.'

Toothache

'A travelling healer demonstrating the extraction of a tooth from the mouth of a woman patient, before a crowd of onlookers.'

Venereal Disease

'A man in bed suffering from syphilis, amidst a busy domestic scene, 1600.'

Pregnancy

'Engraving showing the gravid womb and its blood supply on the left, and a child in the womb on the right, 1676.'

Treatments

'Constipation was often relieved using a clyster or liquid enema delivered by syringes such as these. Note the different types of syringe, for the penis, the vagina, and the rectum.'

'A doctor administers a clyster to a greedy little boy who is laying across his mother's lap, his two siblings watch the scene with amusement.'

'Illustration showing the position of two cupping glasses on the buttocks of a gentleman, 1694.'

'"Lancets and flambets": Instruments for blood-letting, 1612.'

'Ointment jar. With the name of Stewart, 12, 13, Broad Street, Manufactory. Late seventeenth to early eighteenth century.'

'A page from Susan Tully, Lady Hoare's "Book of Receipts for Cookery and Pastry & c" containing treatment on the following: 'For a Rheum in the Eyes', 'For a Whitelow or Fellon', 'For a Pain in the Side' and 'For them that can't make Water' Eighteenth Century.'

Bibliography

Manuscript Primary Sources

Bodleian Library, MD.Rawl.D.78, Elizabeth Delaval, 'Meditations and Prayers'.

British Library, MS Sloane 4076, f. 224-5.

Cambridge Archive, K17/C/1, 'Earl of Halifax letter to the Bishop John Moore'.

Derbyshire Record Office, D3155/C/46, Sir Arthur Kaye.

Royal College of Physicians, MS 654, 'Sarah Wigges, her Booke'.

Somerset Heritage Centre, DD/X/HKN/1, Dr John Westover his journal 1686-1700.

Staffordshire Record Office, 5350, Dr Wilkes Journal.

Wellcome Library, MS 1026, Lady Ayscough recipe book.

Wellcome Library, MS 1548, Mary Chantrell.

Wellcome Library, MS 2535, Elizabeth Godfrey.

Wellcome Library, MS 3009, Elizabeth Jacob.

Wellcome Library, MS 3712, Elizabeth Okeover.

Wellcome Library, MS 3724, Sir Thomas Osborne recipe book.

Wellcome Library, MS 2990, Bridget Hyde's book.

Wellcome Library, MS 1511, Mrs Carr's book.

Wellcome Library, MS 373, Jane Jackson c.1642.

Wellcome Library, MS 7721, English recipe book, 17th-18th century.

Wellcome Library, MS 4338, Johanna Saint John.

Wellcome Library, MS 160, Anne Brumwich.

Wellcome Library, MS 3107, The recipe book of Edward and Katherine Kidder.

Wellcome Library, MS 5006, Richard Wilkes Observations volume 2.

Printed Primary Sources

[Anon.], *An Account of the Causes of some Particular Rebellious Distempers* (London, 1670).

[Anon.], *An Answer to a Scoffing and Lying Lybell; put forth and privately dispersed under the title of a wonderful account of the curing the kings-evil, by Madam Fanshaw the Duke of Monmouth's Sister* (London, 1681).

[Anon.], *Aristoteles Master-Piece; or, The Secrets of Generation Displayed in All the Parts* (London, 1684).

[Anon.], *The Ceremonies us'd in the time of King Henry VII for the Healing of them that be diseas'd with the Kings evil* (London, 1686).

[Anon.], *An Essay on the Ancient and Modern use of Physical Necklaces for Childrens Teeth, with a Treatise on the Tooth-ach: and Hollow Rotten Teeth* (London, 1726).

[Anon.], *Choice and Rare Experimented Receipts in Physick and Chirurgery* (London, 1675).

[Anon.], *The County-mans physician* (London, 1680).

[Anon.], *In Exeter-street, near Exeter-change in the Strand, next door to the Black-Moors-Head, liveth a gentlewoman* (London, 1680?).

[Anon.], *The Historie of the Life and Reigne of that Famous Princesse, Elizabeth* (London, 1634).

[Anon.], *The Lady's Companion: Or, an infallible guide to the fair sex* (London, 1743).

[Anon.], *The London jilt, or, the Politick whore shewing all the artifices and stratagems which the ladies of pleasure make use of for the intreaguing and decoying of men* (London, 1683).

[Anon.], *A Mechanical Enquiry into the Nature, Causes, Seat, and Cure of the Diabetes* (Oxford, 1745).

[Anon.], *Orders Conceived and Published by the Lord Major and Aldermen of the City of London, concerning the Infection of the Plague* (London, 1665).

[Anon.] *The Plagues approved Physitian* (London, 1665).

[Anon.], *The Poore-mans Plaster-box. Furnished with diverse Excellent Remedies for sudden Mischances, and usuall infirmities, which happen to Men, Women, and Children in this Age* (London, 1634).

[Anon.], *The Practical Scheme of Secret Injuries and Broken Constitutions* (London, 1719).

[Anon.], *The Secret Patient's Diary: Also the Gout and Weakness Diaries. Being Each A Practical Journal or Scheme from Day to Day, of these Disorders, whilst a Person has the Secret Disease, or the Gout, or Rheumatism, or a Gleet upon them …* (London, 1725).

[Anon.], *A True and Wonderful Account of a Cure of the Kings-Evil, by Mrs. Fanshaw, Sister to his Grace the Duke of Monmouth* (London, 1681).

[Anon.], *The Whole Aphorismes of Great Hippocrates Prince of Physicians* (London, 1610).

Adams, Thomas, *The blacke devil or the apostate. Together with the wolfe worrying the lambes* (London, 1615).

Allen, Charles, *Curious observations in that difficult part of chirurgery, relating to the teeth* (Dublin, 1687).

Andry, Nicolas, *An Account of the Breeding of Worms in Human Bodies* (London, 1701).

Aristotle [pseudo], *The Problemes of Aristotle with other Philosophers and Phi sitions* (Edinburgh, 1595).

Arrais, Edward Madeira, *A Physical Account of the Tree of Life* (London, 1683).

Astruc, John, *A treatise of the Venereal Disease,* translated by S. Chapman, surgeon (London, 1755).

Aubrey, John, *Miscellanies upon the following subjects* (London, 1696).

Bacon, Roger, *The Cure of Old Age and preservation of youth* (London, 1683).

Baley, Walter, *Two Treatises Concerning the Preservation of Eye-sight* (London, 1616).

Barbette, Paul, *Thesaurus Chirurgiae: The Chirurgical and Anatomical Works of Paul Barbette* (London, 1687).

Barret, Robert, *A Companion for Midwives, Child-Bearing Women, and Nurses Directing them How to Perform their Respective Offices* (London, 1699).

Barrough, Philip, *Methode of Physicke* (London, 1583).

Bayfield, Robert, *Enchiridion Medicum* (London, 1655).

Boulton, Richard, *Physico-chyrurgical treatises of the Gout, the Kings-evil and the Lues Venerea* (London, 1715).

Boyle, Robert, *Medicinal Experiments or a Collection of Choice and Safe Remedies* (London, 1693).

Browne, John, *The Surgeons Assistant. In which is plainly discovered the True Origin of most Diseases. Treating particularly of the Plague, French Pox, Leprosie, &c* (London, 1703).

Brunschwig, Hieronymus von, *The Vertuose boke of distyllacyon of the waters,* trans. Laurence Andrew (London, 1527).

Bullein, William, *Bulleins Bulwarke of Defence Against all Sicknesse, Soarenesse, and Woundes* (London, 1579).

Buchan, William, *Domestic Medicine: Or a treatise on the prevention and cure of diseases* (London, 1772).

C., R., *Advertisement. The Book of Direction* (London, 1661?).

C., T., *An Hospitall for the Diseased* (London, 1579).

Cavendish, Margaret, Duchess of Newcastle, *Ground of Natural Philosophy* (London, 1668).

Chamberlayne, Thomas, *The Compleat Midwifes Practice* (London, 1656).

Cheselden, William, *A Treatise on the High Operation for the Stone* (London, 1723).

Clark, Henry, *His Grace The Duke of Monmouth Honoured in His Progress in the West of England in an Account of a most Extraordinary Cure or the Kings Evil* (London, 1680).

Clowes, Willian, *A Briefe and Necessary Treatise touching the cure of the disease called Morbus Gallicus* (London, 1585).

Cockburn, William, *The Symptoms, Nature, Cause, and Cure of Gonorrhoea*, 2nd edn (London, 1715).

--- *Sea diseases: or, a treatise of their nature, causes and cure* (London, 1736).

Cotgrave, Randle, *A Dictionarie of the French and English Tongues* (London, 1611).

Culpeper, Nicholas, *A Directory for Midwives; or, a Guide for Women, in their Conception, Bearing, and Suckling their children* (London, 1651).

--- *Pharmacopoeia Londinensis: Or the London Dispensatory* (London, 1653).

--- *Culpeper's Directory for Midwives: or, A Guide for Women* (London, 1662).

--- *The English Physitian Enlarged* (London, 1669).

De la Vauguion, *A Compleat body of Chirurgical Operations Containing the Whole Practice of Surgery, with Observations and Remarks on each case* (London, 1699).

De le Boe, Franciscus, *Dr. Franciscus de le Boe Sylvius of Childrens diseases* (London, 1682).

Defoe, Daniel, *A Journal of the Plague Year: being observations or memorials, of the most remarkable occurrences, as well publick as private, which happened in London during the last great visitation in 1665* (London, 1722).

Donne, John, *Poems by J. D. with elegies on the Author's Death* (London, 1633).

Fage, John, *Speculum Ægrotorum* (London, 1606).

Forster, William, *A Treatise on the Causes of most Diseases Incident to Human Bodies, and the Cure* (Leeds, 1745).

Francis Herring, *A Modest Defence of the caveat given to the wearers of impoisoned amulets* (London, 1604).

Freind, John, *Emmenologia*, trans. by Thomas Dale (London, 1729).

Fuller, Thomas, *Pharmacopoeia Extemporanea* (London, 1730).

Gerard, John, *The Herball or Generall Historie of Plantes* (London, 1633).

Gibson, Thomas, *The Anatomy of Human Bodies Epitomized* (London, 1682).

Groenevelt, Joannes, *Arthritology, or a Discourse of the Gout* (London, 1691).

Guillemeau, Jacques, *A Worthy Treatise of the Eyes*, trans by Anthony Hunton (London, 1587).

Harper, Thomas, *Gutta Podagrica a treatise of the gout* (London, 1633).

Hartman, G., *True Preserved and Restorer of Health: being a Choice Collection of Select and Experienced Remedies* (London, 1682).

Harvey, Gideon, *Little Venus Unmask'd, or, A perfect discovery of the French pox* (London, 1670).

Heinsius, Daniel, *Laus Pediculi: or An Apologeticall Speech*, trans. by James Guitard (London, 1634).

Hobbs, Stephen, *Margarita Chyrurgica: Containing A Compendious Practise of Chyrurgie. Selected and translated, out of the Works of the most Famous Physitions, and Chyrurgions of this Age* (London, 1610).

Holland, Philemon, *The Historie of the World, commonly called The Natural Historie of C. Plinius Secundis* (London, 1601).

Kellwaye, Simon, *A defensatiue against the plague contayning two partes or treatises* (London, 1593).

Kemp, W., *A Brief Treatise of the nature, causes, signes, preservation from, and cure of the pestilence* (London, 1665).

Lanfranc of Milan, *A Most Excellent and Learned Work of Chirurgerie* (London, 1565).

La Calmette, François de., *Riverius Reformatus: or the modern Riverius; containing the modern practice of physick. Much like that of Riverius* (London, 1713).

Le Clerc, Charles Gabriel, *The Compleat Surgeon: or the whole art of surgery explain'd* (London, 1696).

Le Clerc, Daniel, *The History of Physick, or, an account of the Rise and Progress of the Art* (London, 1699).

Levnius Lemnius, *The Secret Miracles of Nature* (London, 1658).

Lodge, Thomas, *A Treatise of the Plague containing the Nature, Signes, and Accidents of the Same* (London, 1603).

Lovell, Robert, *Pambotanologia sive Enchiridion Botanicum. Or a Compleat Herball* (Oxford, 1659).

Lower, Richard, *Dr. Lowers, and several other eminent physicians receipts* (London, 1700).

Lupton, Thomas, *A Thousand Notabale Things, of Sundry Sortes* (London, 1579).

Lyte, Henry, *A Nievve Herball, or Historie of Plantes* (London, 1578).

Johnston, Robert, *Enchiridion Medicum, or, a manual of physick* (London, 1684).

Jonstonus, Joannes, *The Idea of Practical Physick in Twelve Books* (London, 1657).

Markham, Gervase, *The English Huswife* (London, 1615).

Marsh, A., *The Ten Pleasures of Marriage Relating all the Delights and Contentments that are Mask'd Under the Bands of Matrimony* (London, 1682).

Marten, John, *A True and Succinct Account of the Venereal Disease* (London 1706).

--- *A Treatise of all the Degrees and Symptoms of the Venereal Disease in both Sexes*, 6th edn (London, 1708).

--- *The Attila of the Gout* (London, 1713).

Massaria, Alessandro, *De Morbis Fœmineis, the Womans Counsellour: or, The Feminine Physitian* (London, 1657).

Maubray, John, *The Female Physician Containing all the Diseases Incident to that Sex in Virgins, Wives and Widows* (London, 1724).

Maurice Tobin, *A True Account of the Celebrated Secret of Mr. Timothy Beaghan lately Killed at the Five Bells Tavern in the Strand, Famous for Curing the King's-Evil* (London, 1697).

Mauriceau, François, *The diseases of women with child, and in child-bed* (London, 1672).

Maynwaring, Everard, *Morbus polyrhizos et polymorphœus, a Treatise of the Scurvy* (1665).

Miller, Joseph, *Botanicum officinale; or a compendious herbal: giving an account of all such plants as are now used in the practice of physick* (London, 1722).

Moyle, John, *An Abstract of Sea-Chirurgery* (London, 1686).

Norford William, *An essay on the General Method of treating Cancerous Tumours* (London, 1753).

O'Dowde, Thomas, *The Poor Man's Physician* (London, 1665).

Oldys, William, *Observations on the cure of William Taylor, the blind boy of Ightham, in Kent* (London, 1753).

Ovington, J., *An Essay upon the Nature and Qualities of Tea* (London, 1699).

P., E., *The New World of English Words: or, a general dictionary* (London, 1658).

Pare, Ambroise, *The Workes of that Famous Chirurgion Ambrose Parey* (London, 1634).

Pechey, John, *A Collection of Chronical Diseases, viz. The Colick, The Bilous Colick: Hysterick Diseases: The Gout: and the Bloody Urine from the Stone in the Kidnies* (London, 1692). .

--- *The Store-house of Physical Practice* (London, 1695).

--- *The Compleat Midwife's Practice* (London, 1698).

Peachi, John, *Some Observations made upon the Herb called Perigua, Imported from the Indies shewing its admirable virtues in curing the diabetes* (London, 1694).

––– *Some Observations made upon the Calumba Wood* (London, 1694).

––– *Some Observations made upon the Malabar Nutt, imported from the Indies* (London, 1694).

––– *Some Observations made upon the Mexico Seeds imported from the Indies* (London, 1695).

Pemell, Robert, *De Morbis Puerorum, or, A Treatise of The Diseases of Children; With Their Causes, Signs, Prognosticks, and Cures, for the benefit of such as do not understand the Latine Tongue, and very useful for all such as are House-keepers, and have Children* (London, 1653).

Perry, Charles, *A treatise of diseases in General. Wherein the true causes, natures, and essences of all the principal diseases incident to the human body, are ... explain'd* (London, 1741) .

Peter, Charles, *Description of the Venereal Disease declaring the causes, signs, effects and cure thereof* (London, 1678).

Philips, George, *A problem concerning the gout in a letter to Sir John Gordon* (London, 1691).

Physician, *A Rational Account of the Natural Weaknesses of Women* (London, 1716).

Pierce, Robert, *Bath Memoirs; or Observations in Three and Forty Years Practice; at the Bath, what Cures have been there wrought* (Bristol, 1697).

Plat, Hugh, *Certaine philosophical preparations of foode and beverage for sea-men, in their long voyages* (London, 1607).

Platter, Felix, *Platerus Golden Practice of Physick* (London, 1664).

[Pope XXI], *The Treasury of Healthe* (London, 1553).

Ramazzini, Bernardino, *A Treatise of the Diseases of Tradesmen* (London, 1705).

Rivière, Lazare, *The Practice of Physick in Seventeen Books*, translated by Nicholas Culpeper and others (London, 1655) .

Rowley, William, *A Practical Treatise on the Diseases of the Breasts of Women* (London, 1772).

Ruscelli, Girolamo, *The Seconde Parte of the Secrets of Maister Alexis of Piemont* (London, 1568).

S., J., *Paidōn nosēmata· = or Childrens diseases* (London, 1664).

Sadler, John, *The Sicke Womans Private Looking-Glasse* (London, 1636).

Salmon, William, *Iatrica, seu, Praxis medendi: The Practice of Curing being a Medicinal History* (London, 1681).

––– *Synopsis Medicinæ* (London, 1671).

––– *Family Dictionary* (London, 1695).

––– *Pharmacopoeia Londinensis: or, a new London dispensatory* (London, 1707).

Scaife, William and Isabel, *A short relation of some words and expressions that were spoken by Barbara scaife in time of her sickness* (London, 1686).

Sennert, Daniel, Nicholas Culpeper and Abdiah Cole, *Two Treatises* (London, 1660).

Sermon, William, *A friend to the sick, or, The honest Englishman's preservation* (London, 1673).

Shakespeare, William, *His true chronicle historie of the life and death of King Lear and his three daughters* (London, 1608).

Sharp, Jane, *The Midwives Book, or the Whole Art of Midwifery Discovered* (London, 1671).

Simpson, William, *An Historical Account of the Wonderful Cures wrought by Scarbrough Spa* (London, 1680).

Stubbe, Henry, *An Epistolary Discourse Concerning Phlebotomy* (London, 1671).

Stukeley, William, *Of the Gout: in Two Parts* (London, 1734).

Sydenham, Thomas, *The Compleat Method of Curing almost all Diseases to which is added an exact description of their several symptoms* (London, 1694).

Talbor, Robert, *Pyretologia, a Rational Account of the Cause & Cure of Agues* (London, 1672).

Tanner, John, *The hidden treasures of the art of physic* (London, 1659).

Thompson, George, *Galeno-pale A Chymical Trial of the Galenists* (London, 1665).

Trye, Mary, *Medicatrix, or The Woman Physician* (London, 1675).

Turner, Daniel, *De Morbis Cutaneis: A Treatise of Diseases Incident to the Skin* (London, 1723).

––– *The Ancient Physician's Legacy Impartially Surveyed* (London, 1733).

Turner, Robert, *Botanologia* (London, 1664).

Venette, Nicolas, *Conjugal Love Reveal'd; in the Nightly Pleasures of the Marriage Bed* (London, 1720).

Vicary, Thomas, *The English-mans Treasure* (London, 1641).

––– *The Surgions Directorie, for Young Practitioners, in Anatomie, Wounds, and Cures* (London, 1651).

von Hutten, Ulrich, *Of the Wood called Guaiacum* (London, 1539).

Wallace, Thomas, *The Farrier's and Horseman's complete dictionary* (London, 1759).

Ward, William, trans. *The Seconde Part of the Secretes of Master Alexis of Piemont* (London, 1560).

Willis, Thomas, *Dr. Willis's practice of physick being the whole works of that renowned and famous physician wherein most of the diseases belonging to the body of man are treated of* (London, 1684).

--- *The London Practice of Physick* (London, 1685).

--- *An Essay of the Pathology of the Brain and Nervous Stock in which Convulsive Diseases are Treated of Being the Work of Thomas Willis*, trans. by Samuel Pordage (London, 1681).

Willughby, Percival, *Observations in Midwifery*, ed by Henry Blenkinsop (Warwick, 1863).

Wiseman, Richard, *Severall Chirurgical Treatises* (London, 1686).

Woolley, Hannah, *The Accomplish'd Lady's Delight* (London, 1675).

Newspapers

British Apollo 1709 No. 2. 2/2 .

Common Sense or The Englishman's Journal (London, England), Saturday, May 22, 1742; Issue 275.

Daily Courant (London, England), Wednesday, February 26, 1707; Issue 1518.

Daily Journal (London, England), Monday, May 11, 1724; Issue 1031.

Middlesex Journal or Chronicle of Liberty, London, England, Saturday, august 24, 1771, issue 375.

Poor Robins Intelligence (London, England), April 25, 1676 - May 1, 1676.

Editions

Adcock, Rachel, Sara Read, and Anna Ziomek, eds., *Flesh and Spirit: An Anthology of Seventeenth-century Women's Writing* (Manchester: Manchester University Press, 2014).

Beresford, John (ed.), *James Woodforde: the diary of a country parson 1758-1802 with an introduction by Ronald Blythe* (Norwich: Canterbury, 1999).

Clegg, James, *The Diary of James Clegg of Chapel en le Frith, 1708-1755*, part 1, ed by Vanessa S Doe (Matlock: Derbyshire Record Society, 1978).

De Beer, E. S. (ed.), *The Diary of John Evelyn* (London: Oxford University Press, 1959).

Dewhurst, Kenneth, *John Locke Physician and Philosopher: A Medical Biography with an edition of the medical notes in his journals* (London: The Wellcome Historical Medical Library, 1963).

Hobby, Elaine (ed.) Raynalde, Thomas, *The Birth of Mankind; otherwise Named the Woman's Book* (Aldershot: Ashgate, 2009).

Hockliffe, E. (ed.), *The Diary of the Rev. Ralph Josselin 1616-1683* edited for the Royal Historical Society Camden Third Series, vol. xv (London, 1908).

Hunter, Michael, and Annabel Gregory (eds), *An Astrological Diary of the Seventeenth Century: Samuel Jeake of Rye 1652-1699* (Oxford: Clavendon Press, 1988).

Hutton, Sarah, *The Conway Letters edited by Marjorie Hope Nicolson* (Oxford: Clarendon, 1992).

Lane, Joan, *John Hall and his Patients: The Medical Practice of Shakespeare's Son-in-Law* (Stratford: The Shakespeare Birthplace Trust, 1996).

Moody, Joanna, (ed.), *The Private Correspondence of Jane Lady Cornwallis Bacon 1613-1644* (London and Cranbury NJ, 2003).

Prior, Matthew, (ed.) John Wilmot, Earl of Rochester, '*Tunbridge-Wells*. By the Earl of Rochester, June 30. 1675' in *State-poems; continued from the time of O. Cromwel, to this present year 1697* (London, 1697).

Searle, Arthur (ed.), *Barrington Family Letters 1628-1632* Camden Fourth Series, Volume 28 (London, 1983).

Smith, Thomas, (ed.), *Poetica Erotica: A Collection of Rare and Curious Amatory Verse* (New York: Boni and Liveright, 1921–22) [via www.bartleby.com].

Wheatley, Henry B. (ed), *The Diary of Samuel Pepys. M.A. F.R.S. Clerk of the acts and Secretary to the admiralty. Transcribed from the shorthand manuscript in the Pepysian library Magdalene College Cambridge by the rev. Mynors bright m.a. Late fellow and president of the college* (London, 1893).

Online Sources

http://classics.mit.edu/Hippocrates/sacred.html 'On the Sacred Disease'.

http://earlymodernmedicine.com A blog on medicine and gender.

http://eebo.chadwyck.com 'Early English Books Online' [Subscription required].

http://gale.cengage.co.uk 'Eighteenth Century Collections Online' [Subscription required].

Greengrass, M., Leslie M., and Hannon, M. (2013) *The Hartlib Papers*. Published by HRI Online Publications, Sheffield [available at http://hrionline.ac.uk/hartlib].

http://www.obgyn.net For statistics on molar pregnancy rates.

http://www.oldbaileyonline.org 'The Proceedings of the Old Bailey 1676-1913'.

Further Reading

Barry, Jonathan, *The Tudor and Stuart Town 1530-1688: A Reader in English Urban History* (London and New York: Routledge, 2014; 1990).

Brogan, Stephen, *The Royal Touch in early modern England. Politics, Medicine and Sin* (Woodbridge: Boydell & Brewer, 2015).

— 'The Royal Touch', *History Today* 61.2 (2011).

Dobson, Mary J., *Contours of Death and Disease in Early Modern England* (Cambridge: Cambridge University Press, 2002).

Davies, Owen, and Francesca Matteoni, 'A virtue beyond all medicine': The Hanged Man's Hand, Gallows Tradition and Healing in Eighteenth- and Nineteenth-century England', *Social History of Medicine,* 28.4 (2015), 686-705.

Elmer, Peter, *The Miraculous Conformist: Valentine Greatrakes, the Body Politic, and the Politics of Healing in Restoration Britain* (Oxford: Oxford University Press, 2013).

Evans, Jennifer, *Aphrodisiacs, Fertility and Medicine in Early Modern England* (Woodbridge: Boydell & Brewer, 2014).

Furdell, Elizabeth Lane, *Fatal Thirst: Diabetes in Britain until Insulin* (Leiden: Brill, 2009).

Gentilcore, David, *Medical Charlatanism in early modern Italy* (Oxford: Oxford, University Press, 2006).

Gratzer, Walter, *Terrors of the Table: The Curious History of Nutrition* (Oxford: Oxford University Press, 2005).

Heffernan, Troy, 'Protecting England and its Church: Lady Anne and the death of Charles Stuart', *The Seventeenth Century*, 31.3 (2016) 57-70 .

Hoffmann-Axthelm, Walter, *History of Dentistry* (Chicago: Quintessence Publishing Company, 1981).

Jones, Colin, 'The King's Two Teeth', *History Workshop Journal*, 65.1, (2008), 79-95.

Jutte, Robert, 'Ageing and Body Image in the Sixteenth Century: Hermann Weinsberg's (1518-97) Perception of the Ageing Body', *European History Quarterly*, 18 (1988).

King, Helen, *Midwifery, Obstetrics and the Rise of Gynaecology: The Uses of a Sixteenth-Century Compendium* (Aldershot: Ashgate, 2007).

Lindeman, Mary *Medicine and Society in Early Modern Europe* (Cambridge: Cambridge University Press, 2010).

Mortimer, Ian, 'The Rural Medical Marketplace in Southern England c. 1570-1720', in *Medicine and the Market in England and its Colonies, c. 1450-c. 1850*, edited by Mark S. R. Jenner and Patrick Wallis (Palgrave: Basingstoke, 2007), pp. 69-87.

Mukherjee, Siddhartha, *The Emperor of All Maladies: A Biography of Cancer* (London: Fourth Estate, 2011).

Munkhoff, Richelle, 'Searchers of the Dead: Authority, Marginality and the Interpretation of Plague in England 1574-1665', *Gender & History*, vol. 11.1 (1999), 1-29.

Newton, Hannah, *The Sick Child in early modern England, 1580-1720* (Oxford: Oxford University Press, 2012).

Pelling, Margaret, *The Common Lot: Sickness, Medical Occupations and the Urban Poor in early modern England* (London and New York: Longman, 1998).

Pietzman, Steven J., *Dropsy, Dialysis, Transplant: a short history of failing kidneys* (Baltimore: The Johns Hopkins University Press, 2007).

Pollock, Linda, *With Faith and Physic: The Life of a Tudor Gentlewoman Lady Grace Mildmay, 1552–1620* (New York: Collins and Brown, 1993).

Porter, Roy and Lesley Hall, *The Facts of Life: The Creation of Sexual Knowledge in Britain, 1650-1950* (New Haven and London: Yale university Press, 1995).

Porter, Roy, '"Laying Aside Any Private Advantage": John Marten and Venereal Disease', in *The Secret Malady: Venereal Disease in Eighteenth-Century Britain and France* (Lexington, Ken: The University Press of Kentucky, 1996).

--- and G. S. Rousseau, *Gout: the Patrician Malady* (London and New Haven: Yale University Press, 1998).

Read, Sara, *Menstruation and the Female Body in Early Modern England* (Basingstoke: Palgrave, 2013).

Rowland, Beryl, ed., *Medieval Woman's Guide to Health: The First English Gynaecological Handbook* (London: Kent University Press, 1981).

Sarasohn, Lisa T., 'The Microscopist as Voyeur: Margaret Cavendish's Critique of Experimental Philosophy', in *Challenging Orthodoxies: the social and cultural worlds of early modern women*, eds Sigrun Haude, Melinda S Zook (Farnham: Ashgate, 2014).

Shail, Andrew and Gillian Howe, eds., *Menstruation: A Cultural History* (London: Palgrave Macmillan, 2005).

Siena, Kevin, *Venereal Disease, Hospitals and the Urban Poor: London's 'Foul Wards' 1600-1800* (Rochester: University of Rochester Press, 2004).

Skuse, Alanna, *Constructions of Cancer in Early Modern England: Ravenous Natures* (Basingstoke: Palgrave, 2015).

Townend, B. R., 'The Story of the Tooth-worm', *Bulletin of the History of Medicine* 15 (1944), 37–58.

Wallis, Patrick, 'Exotic Drugs and English Medicine: England's Drug Trade, c. 1550-c.1800, *Social History of Medicine*, 25.1 (2012), 20–46.

——'Plagues, Morality and the Place of medicine in early modern England', *The English Historical Review*, 121/4 (2006), 1-24.

Zell, Michael, *Early Modern Kent 1540-1640* (Woodbridge: The Boydell Press, 2000).

Index

Adulteration of drugs, 66
Advertisements, xx, 5, 26, 27, 32, 35, 36, 71, 91, 117, 157–8, 159
Ageing, xiv, 18, 20, 25, 36, 39, 72, 88, 122, 128
Agrippa, Henry Cornelius, 15
Alcohol, xxii, 4, 5, 14, 17, 18, 21, 22, 25, 42, 44, 45,47, 53, 54, 65, 66, 69, 75, 79, 83, 86, 87, 106, 115, 116, 132, 139, 150, 160
Allen, Charles, 36
Americas, The, 64
Amulets, 15, 64, 105, 149–50
Anne, Queen, 51,107, 119
Archer, Anne, 62
Archer, Isaac, 23, 62
Aristotle, x, xix
Army see Soldiers, 152
Astrology, xv–xvi, 60
Astruc, John, 154
Aubrey, John, 120
Avicenna, 121

Bacon, Francis, Viscount St Alban, xx
Barbette, Paul, 28, 51, 107
Barrington, Lady Joan, xxiii, 21, 50, 86
Barrough, Phillip, 3, 4, 14, 43, 45, 49, 67, 80
Bayfield, Robert, 157
Beauty see also disfigurement, 36, 119, 125, 154–5
Bellini, Lorenzo, xix
Bills of Mortality, xxiv–xxv, 35, 43, 72, 73, 80, 100–101
Blood, x, xi, xii, xviii, 5, 7, 11, 12, 17, 33, 34, 36, 41, 42, 43, 46, 51, 64, 67, 68, 72, 74, 77, 79, 81, 86, 93, 94, 111, 121–2, 124, 128, 129,130–1,133, 135, 137, 146, 156, 158
    Circulation of, xi, 79
    Humour, x, xi, 112, 117, 121
    Letting, xviii, 44, 62, 63, 82, 124, 128, 130–1
    Menstrual, xii, 15, 68, 121, 122, 128, 139–40, 146
Boyle, Robert, 2, 30, 69, 116

Boyle, Roger, first earl of Orrery, 3, 90
Bread, 5, 6, 21, 24, 51, 77, 95, 105, 112
Breast milk, 41, 122
Brunschwig, Hieronymus von, 39
Bunworth, Richard, 152

Cambridgeshire, 47, 66
Caudle, 85,
Celsus, Aulus Cornelius, xvii
Chamberlayne, Thomas, 145
Charles II, King, xviii, 66, 108
Charms see amulets
Chemical Medicine, xv, xvii–xviii, 12, 39, 52, 79, 103, 117, 161
Chesleden, William, 56
Childbirth, xxv, 123, 137, 147, 150
Childhood illness, 13, 14, 20, 35, 40–1, 46, 52, 94–6, 119, 120, 122, 155–6
Choler (humour), x, xv, 7, 40, 43, 45, 47, 61, 69, 86, 129
Clegg, Ann, 143
Clegg, James, 13, 120, 124, 143, 144
Clerc, Charles Gabriel le, 8, 70
Clerc, Daniel le, 28
Cockburn, William, 115–16, 135, 136, 137
Coe, William, 143
Columbus, Christopher, 153
Commonplace book, x
Constantinople, 126
Constitution (Humoral), x, xi, xv, 17, 39, 88, 95, 107, 157
Conway, Lady Anne, Viscountess Conway and Killultagh, 2–3, 7, 9, 90, 109
Cordials, 42, 62, 82, 124, 147
Correspondence, xii, 2, 28, 50, 53–4, 62, 65, 86, 87, 126, 129, 139, 148, 151, 159
Cotgrave, Randle, 27
Cowper, Lady Sarah, née Holled, 20, 25
Crisis, 7, 45, 49
Crooke, Helkiah, 19
Culpeper, Nicholas, xiii–xiv, xv, xxiii, xxiv, 10, 12, 31, 46, 69, 77, 86, 131, 133, 140, 149

D'ewes, Sir Simonds, 139
Death, causes of, xxiv–xxvi
Delaval, Lady Elizabeth, née Livingstone, 33
Diagnostic tests, 8, 49, 67, 75–6, 140, 157
Diemerbroeck, Isbrand van, 57, 80, 81, 96
Disfigurement, 119, 156
Dissection, xxi, 80
Domestic Medicine, xxi, xxiii, xxvi, 5–6, 8, 21, 25, 30, 32, 42, 45, 48, 64, 77, 83, 95, 105, 106, 117–18, 150, 157, 161
Donne, John, 91, 93
Drunkenness *see* alcohol
Dury, John, 28

Earthworms, 6, 45, 47, 83, 96, 118, 161
Elizabeth I, Queen, xv, 44, 108, 119, 123, 124
Emetic *see* vomit
Emotions (as a cause of disease), xv, 51, 148, 149
Enema, 38, 40, 95, 124
Environment, 61, 104
Ettmüller, Michael, 41, 74, 76, 82, 83
Essex, 47, 61, 66
Evelyn, John, 17, 39, 40, 52, 63, 80, 97, 119–20
Exercise, x, 14, 51, 63, 86, 90, 130, 134
Experimentation, xi, xviii, xix–xx, 97
    Drug trials, 65, 66, 116,117

Fage, John, x–xi
Fernel, Jean François, 121, 157
Fish, 14, 24, 87, 104
Forster, William, 134, 137
Fracastoro, Girolamo, 122
Fraud (feigning illness), 15
Freind, John, xix, 128
Fumigation, 33, 92, 104, 158

Galen, Claudius, x, xi, xii, xiii, xiv, xix, 4, 18, 38, 73, 121
Gender,
    Bodies xi–xiii, 139, 140
Gerard, John, 33
Gibson, Thomas, xi
God, xvi–xviii, xx, 5, 23, 33, 35, 40, 47, 52, 60, 62, 63, 66, 71, 72, 92, 98, 99, 108, 110, 112, 120, 138, 139, 143, 149, 153
Greatrakes, Valentine, 3, 109–110
Guillemeau, Jacques, 23, 25

Hall, John, xvii, 17, 39, 40, 44, 54–5, 67, 82–3, 95–6, 97, 122, 124, 125, 137, 151

Handbills *see also* advertisements, xx, 5, 35, 117
Hartlib, Samuel, 27, 28, 53–4, 91, 96
Harvey, William, xi, 2
Heinsius, Daniel, 92–3
Helmont, Jean Baptist van, xvii, 21, 79, 80
Helmontians, xvii, 113
Henry VIII, King, xxii, 30, 140
Herbals, 5, 10, 34, 47, 69, 117
Hippocrates, x, xii, xix, 7, 10, 11, 67, 84, 131, 161
Hobbs, Stephen, xii
Hoby, Lady Margaret, xx, iii, 38, 138, 142
Hogarth, William, 160
Holland, Philemon, 30, 67, 87
Horoscopes *see* Astrology
Howard, Lady Katherine, Countess of Suffolk, 119
Hygiene,
    Dental, 30
    Personal, 91, 92

Infanticide, 123
Inoculation (and variolation), 125–6
Irregular healers, xxi, xx, 5, 103
Isham, Elizabeth, 130
Itinerant healers, xxi, 33, 56, 126

James I and IV, King, xxii, 109
James II, King, 108
Jeake, Samuel, 31, 32, 60, 62
Jesuits' Powder (cinchona), 64–6
Johnson, Robert, 4, 5, 6, 7, 56
Jonson, Benjamin, xv, 133, 152
Jonstonus, Joannes (or John Jonston), 12, 45, 74

Kaye, Sir Arthur, 148–9
Kellwaye, Simon, 121–2, 124
Kent, 29, 61–2, 95
Kitchen Physic *see* domestic medicine

Laxatives, 39, 44, 48, 55, 82, 137, 161
Leeches, xi, 5
Letters *see* Correspondence
Lemnius, Levinus, 4, 18, 154
Libido, 63, 145, 154–5
Locke, John, 6, 14, 18, 21, 25, 29, 32, 55, 63, 65, 89, 149–50
Lodge, Thomas, 103

Lovell, Robert, 5
Luttrell, Narcissus, 73
Lyte, Henry, 10

Markham, Gervase, xxiii, 45
Marriage, xv, 62, 63, 131, 138, 139, 141, 145, 149
Marten, John, 89, 136, 155, 156, 158, 159
Masculinity, xiii
Mason, Simon, xix–xx, 61, 63, 64
Maubray, John, 144–45
Mayerne, Theodore Turquet de, 2
Mead, Richard, 124
Meautys, Lady Anna, 149, 151
Mechanical medicine, xviii–xix, 75, 161
Medical Marketplace, xxi
Melancholy, x, xvi, 43, 45, 62, 67, 114, 129, 134, 135
Menstruation, xii, xix, 15, 44, 68, 86, 121–2, 128, 130, 133, 135, 139, 145
Microscope, 91
Midwifery, xx, 46, 68, 82–3, 131–2, 134, 143, 144, 145, 147
Mildmay, Lady Grace, 14
Miller, Joseph, 46, 47
Milton, John, 24, 28–9
More, Henry, 2, 3, 109–110

Napier, Richard, xvi
Navy, 115, 118
Neutral body, xiii–xiv
Newspapers, 68, 126
    Advertisements in, 157–8
Non–naturals, xiv–xv, 38, 130

O'Dowde, Thomas, xviii, 103, 152, 153, 155–6
Old age see ageing
Old Bailey see also theft, 3, 15, 27, 32, 71, 123, 158
Oldys, William, 25, 29
Ovington, John, 75

Pain, xiii, xxiv, 3, 4, 5, 7, 8, 9, 26, 31, 32, 33, 35, 36, 39, 40, 50, 51, 55, 60, 62, 67, 74, 84, 86, 87–8, 90, 98, 114, 124, 134–5, 137, 141, 143, 149, 155, 156, 157, 160, 161
Pain relief, 5, 32, 89, 90
    Anodyne Necklace, 35
Panaceas, 5, 71, 157
Paracelsus (Theophrasus Aurelius von Honhenheim), xvii–xviii

Paré, Ambroise, 8, 110, 157, 160
Patent medicines, 5, 71–2, 79, 114, 115, 130, 157, 159
Poultice, 95, 112
Peachi, John, 73, 75, 76, 85, 89, 96, 110, 111–12
Pechey, John, 75, 76–7, 88, 131
Pepys, Elizabeth, 31, 32, 35, 91, 138, 142
Pepys, Samuel, 4, 25, 26, 31, 50, 56, 57, 87–8, 91, 92, 94, 101, 102, 113, 138
Perronet, David, 30
Perry, Charles, 74, 77–8
Phlegm (humour), x, xi, 5, 11, 12, 13, 14, 18, 28, 32, 39, 61, 79, 83, 86, 94, 95, 107, 117, 121, 129
Phlebotomy see bloodletting
Pica, 129, 130
Pitcairne, Archibald, xix
Poisons, 43, 65, 105, 158
Powell, Vavasor, 11
Prayer, xvii, 11, 13, 15, 38, 99, 120, 138, 143, 161
Pregnancy, xii, 3, 48, 123, 130, 138–51 passim
Prosthetics,
    Eyes, 27
    Teeth, 36
Prostitutes, 136, 140, 153, 154, 160
Providence, xvi–xvi, 35, 109
Puberty, 13, 128
Purges, xv, 14, 17, 20, 22, 38, 39, 41, 44, 63, 69, 82, 83, 95, 117, 130–1, 132, 137
Purmann, Matthew, 52
Puppy, 89

Quincy, John, 35

Ranelagh, Lady Katherine, 53
Raynalde, Thomas, 133, 140
Recipe Books, 64, 105
    Anne Brumwich, 106, 150–1
    Bridget Hyde, 18, 83
    Elizabeth Godfrey, 42, 77, 118
    Elizabeth Jacob, 32
    Elizabeth Okeover, 5, 150, 151
    Jane Jackson, 32
    Johanna Saint John, 8, 21, 22, 77
    Lady Ayscough, 6, 45, 48, 64, 139
    Mary Chantrell, 6, 83, 95, 118
    Mrs Carr, 21

Mrs Corlyon, 6
Sir Thomas Osborne, 6, 47, 117
Rich, Mary, Countess of Warwick, 88
Rivière, Lazare, 18, 20, 31, 35–6, 51, 52, 56, 129, 130–1, 140–1.
Royal College of Physicians, xvii, xxi, xxiii, 33, 73, 103, 141
Royal Society, xx, 97, 126
Rowley, William, 70–1

Sadler, John, 133, 134, 146
Sailors, 113, 115
Salmon, William, 15, 18, 22, 50, 67, 112, 125, 140
Sanctorius, Santorio, xix
Scaife, Barbara, 120
Seasons, 21, 88, 90, 99
Sennert, Daniel, 80, 86, 139
Sermon, William, 47, 79
Sex see also libido, xiii, 14, 20, 51, 87, 92–3, 131, 134, 145, 152–3, 154–5
Shakespeare, William, xvii, 2, 10, 13, 17, 26, 30, 50
  Plays, 10, 13, 26, 36, 93, 128
Sharp, Jane, xx, 46, 56–7, 68, 72, 122, 128, 131–32, 134, 136, 137, 145, 146, 148, 150
Sidney, Sir Philip, 23
Sight, 7, 23–9, 157
Simpson, William, 48–9, 81
Sloane, Sir Hans, 51, 66, 150
Snails, 55
Society of Apothecaries, xxii, 103
Soldiers, 52, 57, 82, 152–3
Spas, 141
  Bath, 17, 141–2
Bristol, 17, 77–8.
  Scarborough, 48–9
  Tunbridge Wells, 132–3, 141–2
Spectacles, 25–7
St. Thomas' Hospital, 56
Stubbe, Henry, xviii
Suetonius, 10
Suffolk, 47
Surgery, xxii, 9, 126
  Cataracts, 27–9
  Lithotomy (cutting for the stone), 50, 52, 55–7
  Mastectomy, 70
  Trepanation, 3, 7–9

Stools (faeces), 38, 39, 40, 44, 82, 92, 96, 117, 124
Sydenham, Thomas, 63, 65, 90, 122, 132
Sympathy see Doctrine of Signatures, 77

Thaumaturgy, 3, 99, 107, 108–10, 112
Theft, 27
Thompson, George, 52
Throckmorton, Robert, 19
Throckmorton, Jane, 19
Tobacco, xv, 2
Toilet, 38, 123
Transference, 55, 64, 105
Travel see also environment, 3, 6, 17, 32, 52, 63, 66, 77, 85, 103, 106, 109, 115
Tripartite model, xxi–xxii
Trye, Mary, xviii, 103
Turner, Daniel, 76, 92, 93, 94

Urine, 12, 20, 39, 45, 50–7, 74–7, 82, 83, 96, 99, 110, 117, 123, 135, 140

Venette, Nicolas, 155
Vicary, Thomas, 6
Viper, 43
Vomit (including emetics), xi, 4, 8, 9, 14, 22, 39, 42, 44, 61, 62, 82, 89, 92, 96, 97, 99, 147, 148, 151

Waters see Spa, 17, 48, 49, 77, 132
  Distilled, 18, 21, 24, 25, 27, 28, 39, 83, 106, 112, 116, 117, 122, 124, 125
Weather see also seasons, 38, 88
Wet nurse, 154–6
Wigges, Sarah, x, 161
Wilkes, Richard, 53, 55
Willis, Thomas, xix, 2, 10–11, 12, 14, 16, 41, 65, 68, 75
Wilmot, John, Earl of Rochester, 132, 141, 152
Winthrop, John, 53
Wiseman, Richard, xxii, 9, 158
Witchcraft, xxiv, 19, 20, 34
  Alice Samuel, 19, 20
  see also Jane Throckmorton
Wolf (cancer), 67, 68
Woolley, Hannah, 125